FINDING HOPE
ON THE OTHER
SIDE
OF DEPRESSION

FINDING HOPE ON THE OTHER SIDE OF DEPRESSION:

Slogging Through and Breaking Free

Jean Conley Stoddard

Dedication

To my mom.

Support looks like Lillian McCauley Conley.

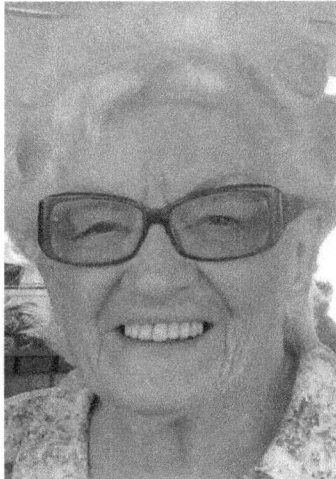

TABLE OF CONTENTS

FOREWORD

One Friday morning in April 2011, my husband Rick and I went on our usual walk through our country-road neighborhood before we each headed off to work. During our then 28-year marriage, it was typical for me to walk Rick to his car, peck his cheek or touch my lips briefly to his before he drove away. This day was no different that way. I then went to my job—an overnight weekend caring for a developmentally disabled adult.

Saturday, Rick was served with divorce papers.

Sunday was Easter.

Correct, I did not leave him kindly. Let's say I was passive-aggressive. I blamed him for another perceived financial stress. But after being apart from Rick for five months, the reality is I couldn't make it on my own. I asked to return, and he took me back.

Two days later, beginning in mid-September 2011, I spent thirty days in three different California psychiatric hospitals diagnosed with clinical depression and anxiety. Most of my hospital experiences were not good, even though Rick visited me every day, accompanied by my mother, who had temporarily moved from Florida during my hospitalization. Mom stayed through December, feeding my undernourished, 109-pound frame and quietly keeping me company.

Family and friends wanted to know what they could do to help. But initially, all that concern didn't matter much to me. Though my hospital experiences were rough, at least for Rick and my mother, the hospitals kept me safe. From whom?

From myself.

This is the story of my long, arduous slog with depression through what truly felt like the valley of the shadow of death—and for a time where I *did* fear evil.[1] (Psalm 23:4)

Today I am thriving and flourishing, for I did eventually find hope on the other side. And my hope is that you will, too!

Chapter 1

DEPRESSION'S HARSH REALITY

The best way to describe my depression was like a category 5, Hurricane Katrina, storm-of-the-mind that pressed and crushed and bore mightily down on my truly troubled and utterly exhausted brain. Its brutal force aimed to obliterate me.

Over time I truly wished I was.

The asteroid I wanted to smash perfectly and exactly on me and my car while driving down the interstate freeway, demolishing us both into extinction, never happened.

A sudden heart attack felt like it would be a welcome death.

And on those rare moments when I finally did fall asleep (though ever-so-briefly), my greatest desire was that I would never wake. Insomnia made each 8-hour nightfall a particularly dark, encumbered, and dreaded form of regular, repeated torment. There's no rest for the wearily depressed!

"I just need the noise (in my brain) to stop," said a fellow depression sufferer to her concerned and frightened mother several years ago.

In truth, the right amygdala, the fight, flight, or freeze part of our brain, is in overdrive with depression. Think of this almond-shaped structure (tiny yet powerful) like a hamster wheel with a poor, exhausted hamster running continually but finding no way to jump off or, better yet, stop altogether.

The thoughts that may be running through a depressed person's mind are often ruminations of the past; therefore, each depressed person suffers from their own unique story. For me, those thoughts included:

- rehashing the unkind way I left Rick
- questioning my choice to leave in the first place
- reliving conversations of family members who were angry at me
- feeling harsh judgment from many
- judging myself as bad
- questioning my decisions on everything
- having an overwhelming desire to isolate

These miserable ruminations melded into one big, lifeless dough ball with no nourishing life force within. No wonder things seemed so dark.

Depression hurts so differently than a broken bone or a bout with the flu. Cancer gets incredible sympathy. Depression? —not usually that kind of support. Physically you seem to look normal to others. Looking normal on the outside makes it easier for some to say to you, "Pick yourself up by the bootstraps." "Shake it off!" "Change direction." "Get on medication" (which may be true). "Just think positive thoughts" (though something can be said for positive thinking). Loved ones indeed are terrified for you but aren't sure what specific things would be helpful.

I was pretty sure that depression was my new, permanent, and eternal reality—that it would never, ever, ever, ever go away. Life felt hopeless. And without hope, what was there, really?

I began to consider other ways to make depression disappear permanently.

I knew there were people who loved me. I knew that my dying by suicide would crush them. I also knew they would feel guilty and wonder what they could have done to help me more. There's a logic to how you know it will affect others. I've lived long enough to have heard many stories of those left behind who suffered deeply after their loved ones ended their lives.

Depression leaves many victims.

But more than anything or more than how anyone would be affected, I SIMPLY WANTED THE PAIN TO GO AWAY!

Yet, even before depression and wanting my life to end, there was anxiety. I look at anxiety as worrying about a future that hasn't happened yet.

I am ten years older than my sister, Julie. We have a shared experience of working jobs during our marriages but not having the burden of being a family breadwinner. We both found that when our jobs got too complicated, the pressure too intense, we had the luxury of quitting each job. (I know many people do not have this luxury or would even call it such.)

I liken the feeling of job pressure to a tea kettle. You turn the burner on to high so the water will boil. The tension in the teapot builds. Though it takes some time, the kettle eventually whistles and the scalding hot water is now ready to use.

That's great for tea-making but not so great for people.

Julie and I could quit our jobs before the kettle whistled—before our anxiety reached the boiling point. It wasn't fun to quit jobs, nor was it easy. Over the years, as it happened with more frequency, the pattern became noticeable and confusing. Still, the quitting-a-job tactic worked at keeping the tea kettle whistle from blowing for many, many years.

Remember that I left Rick over "another perceived financial stress?" Ironically, holding down a job was all on me now. I became my own breadwinner. I paid my monthly cell phone bill, utility bill, and rent. Though I would likely get alimony for a period, two attorneys stated that there would be a time limit. Knowing I had to supply my own health insurance for the rest of my life proved an especially harsh reality.

The tea kettle shrilled long and hard.

It's true that I grew up with an angry father who criticized us kids often, as well as those around him. After he died in 2008, my mom admitted that early in their marriage, she would hide in the closet and cry after receiving each of his verbal tirades. She later learned to give back to him what she got. They bickered a lot. It created unstable footing for me in my life, and I venture to say, within my siblings.

Yes, life can be HARD. Fair or unfair, life is often complicated, tricky, and problematic. Some of us get to slog along the broken, potholed roads of major depressive disorder and generalized anxiety. That slog is an arduous and terrifying journey. Coming out the other side does not seem possible.

In my case, with a whole lot of WORK and plenty of fortunate help, I eventually did come out the other side.

And I hope that you will, too.

Suppose you recognize any degree of this storm-of-the-mind within yourself or others. In that case, my sincere hope for you is that you find the commitment, or faith, or wherewithal, or ability, or courage, or whatever word that works for you to do the tricky work of getting well. You might not believe that you have any degree of momentum to slog forward, but if you are reading this book or a loved one reading this book is helping you, you are still moving through your depression. Early on, I recognized I only needed to take one step at a time—just one. You pick just one thing and do it. Keep doing it for as long as it takes. A day will come when you realize you can now do the next thing.

TAKEAWAYS

1. Can you or your loved one relate to and classify their depression or anxiety as a hurricane? If so, what category is it? (A hurricane's category classifies as 1-5, with five being the most damaging.)[1] This information could be helpful for medical and therapeutic personnel as well as loved ones to know.

2. Others have described their depression or anxiety as a tsunami—a giant wave that washes over them and recedes with time. There are three types of tsunamis—local,

regional, and distant.₂ Still, on a scale of 1-5, with five being the most damaging, a number could be helpful for medical and therapeutic personnel as well as loved ones to know.

3. My friend Hunter who is studying to be a psychotherapist, explained that *depression* is only one word for the thousand other words used to describe each person's unique and varied experience living with mental illness. For Hunter, depression showed up in him as apathy—he could not feel anything. Learning that depression often feels distinctly different within individuals, your depression might not feel like a hurricane, a tsunami, or apathy. It will likely have its own distinct, though distressful, compilation of emotions and sensations within your inner world. Putting words to your depression may be helpful. Using a feeling wheel may aid you in defining with specificity how depression feels.₃

4. This memoir contains several methods that worked for me— one of which was therapy. My Experiential Psychotherapist, Deborah A. (DeBora) Miller, LMFT, who specialized in trauma, threw numerous challenges at me from her psychotherapy toolkit. I would choose the one thing that resonated and could rouse myself to do.

5. In the beginning, getting in my car and driving to the appointment was the only thing I could do.

6. A friend, who reviewed this memoir, found this chapter difficult to read—scary, even. "Depression," she explains, "is the elephant in the room."

7. True, mental illness is challenging to discuss with loved ones, let alone know how to help move toward a solution. My story will provide some helpful ideas, but you will likely realize that your path to mental wellness veers in a different, though beneficial, direction. There are many roads to wellness.

8. There is hope!

Chapter 2

ENTRANCE TO THE VALLEY OF THE SHADOW OF DEATH

To get into a California psychiatric hospital, you must prove you belong there. Going to a regular hospital emergency room, declaring you're exhausted and that you haven't slept for the last month, isn't enough to commit you. No offering of a blessedly prescribed sleeping pill would happen. Dropping weight daily from lack of appetite and a knot in your stomach is not yet of particular concern. None of these reasons signal your need for more support.

Instead, you must sound somewhat weird, loony, and even crazy. The very second you say, "Life isn't worth living." Or "I wish I were dead." the system grants you entry into the "51-50 Club." Section 5150 is the California Legal code for the temporary, involuntary psychiatric commitment of individuals who present a danger to themselves or others due to mental illness.[1] (In Utah, where I currently live, the equivalent law is Utah Human Services Code 62A-15-629.[2] Each state likely has its own version.)

At Psychiatric Hospital 1 (H1), the staff placed me in a room closest to the nurses' station. My female roommate seemed genuinely uneasy and moaned a lot. However, I remember the nurse being kind to her, calling her gently by name, and seeing that she was comfortable in bed. This patient was my roommate for only one night.

Sometime that evening, while in our bedroom, I heard a voice within or perhaps outside me ask, "Do you want to go to the *dark side*?" The *dark side* is a more pleasant name than *hell*, more palatable and less threatening as a Star Wars reference. As I cocked my head slightly to the right, my inquisitive nature simply said, "OK."

With that choice now made, I instantly envisioned a rectangular jewelry box with a silver skeleton key already inserted into the keyhole slot. My response must have caused the key to turn, for the lock clicked loudly, and I felt certain the jewelry box would never open again.

Turning to my left, a vision of hell immediately appeared before me. The scene looked like the messy, dark-grey spectacle depicted in the 1998 movie, *What Dreams May Come*. The murky, charcoal-colored ground showed submerged, freakish, upturned faces. Each sunken soul was barely able to breathe. Their groanings and complaints depicted misery to a vicious degree. I didn't necessarily feel an evil presence in hell. Instead, it was the overwhelming despair and utter hopelessness these struggling beings suffered, in a range of agony I never knew possible, that took me aback.

Eventually, my gaze shifted to the right. If you were with me now as I described what followed, I would smack my hands together loudly while emphatically summarizing, "And from then on, *chaos* followed me *everywhere* I went!"

While in H1, this pandemonium shadowed me for two entire weeks. It next accompanied me in the ambulance for a long weekend at Psychiatric Hospital 2 (H2). And it slithered into a later ambulance, depositing me at Hospital 3 (H3—a combined medical and psychiatric hospital) where I received continued mental monitoring with additional medical support for a bladder infection. Chaos hounded me unmercifully for an entire month!

Chaos looked like psychosis—defined as a severe mental disorder characterized by symptoms, such as delusions or hallucinations that indicate impaired contact with reality.[3] Even now, my memories don't know which parts are true or psychotic. At the time, everything that happened around and inside me seemed real.

Chaos (or psychosis) displayed like this:

- *The change and introduction of new medications proved constant.* For years Armour Thyroid was the *only* prescribed medication I had ever taken. It was for hypothyroidism. Now, in all three hospitals, the anti-psychotic drug Seroquel was added. The 300 mg dose for my 5'4" frame caused my heart to pound repeatedly. Sleep became impossible. Also prescribed were at least four other psychotropic medications.

- *My clothing was no longer in my care.* Though many patients at H1 got their clothes laundered by putting their piles in the hall outside their door, my own clothes weren't. Figuring out the procedure took me a while, but my load stayed outside the door. In the end, my mother occasionally brought laundered clothing from home.

- *I lost control over my life and seemingly my body.* In H1, it was traditional for patients to line up each evening at the dispensary. In front of the staff, I ingested at least five different tablets. Shortly after that, I became very unsteady on my feet. One night while weaving to the bathroom, I fell and hit the back of my head hard. Nurses immediately called an emergency "code blue." The staff monitored me for several hours. However, a proper examination by a medical doctor never happened, and the staff psychiatrist appeared indifferent to my predicament.

- *Socializing and even communicating felt impossible.* Going to the cafeteria and being around others was particularly torturous for me. I knew that I should be talking to the different patients at each table seating. Mostly I felt incapable of putting lucid sentences together—thus, I was often silent. I truly labored in my mind to make coherent small talk.

- *My diet became a weapon.* At that time, I was eating gluten-free. (I have since confirmed that I have one gene for celiac disease.) The H1 cafeteria usually had one type of gluten-free offering. One night, feeling my usual discomfort about going to the cafeteria, I asked to stay behind with those few who took their meals in a room separate from the others. It appeared intentional that the dietician brought up an unpalatable bowl of gluten-free paste (not pasta). I never again asked to stay behind.

- *My brain and mouth didn't work.* At the nurses' station, asking for my shampoo or dental floss (contraband string a person could conceivably harm themselves with) felt confusing and challenging. My tangled tongue asked for these items in slow motion. Conversely, returning items to the nurses' station was equally tricky.

13

- *Memory impairment affected my hygiene.* Though there were specific times to shower, I couldn't remember when those times were, even though laminated instructions were in the bathroom. My personal hygiene in all three hospitals was poor.

- *The entity within would speak to me.* I felt compelled to tell both my husband Rick and the H1 psychiatrist, in what sounded to be a low-pitched and monotonous voice, "I hate you." I sincerely did not hate Rick, but the words came out of my mouth anyway. The H1 psychiatrist? —well, the truth is I did not like her.

- *My affect was blank, quiet, and withdrawn.* I had a felt sense that patients and staff in each location did not like me. On the final day of my release at H1, a man I had previously interacted with purposely stared at me while slowly opening and closing his eyes. His mocking gesture seemed a simulation of something I must have been doing. He finally said, "I am so glad to have met you. You are an example of the kind of person I don't want to be."

- *My mind and body responded poorly to hospital rules.* I felt compelled to obey all hospital policies, so I attended every required class in all three hospitals. Unfortunately, my mind could never do the work. Staff often supplied worksheets to fill out, yet I could not think of one answer to put down—nothing, a totally blank screen. I sensed that the proctor felt the blank pages I returned a display of defiance on my part. It was not.

- *Mental illness made the daily drain of hospital life unbearable.* At H1, being in the larger lecture room with many other patients was tricky. I could sit only for a short while, then erratically, I'd get up and scurry back to my hospital bedroom. I felt shame about being with others when I obviously could not focus. My repeated up-and-down actions embarrassed me, yet I felt compelled to keep doing them.

- *The entity got crazier.* The most psychotic I got was at H1 when I fell obedient to the voice in my head that said aloud to my husband that I needed to kill our newest infant grandchild and two other non-descript babies. Internally, I did not have the wherewithal to do it, nor an authentically genuine desire. I felt impelled, however, to speak those violent words, scaring those around me. I know Rick was deeply disturbed by this talk about killing our grandchild since he still occasionally mentions it to others in my presence.

- *Hospitals can make serious mistakes.* During my brief stay at H2, a female patient with the first name of "Jean" and a last name beginning with the letter "S" received my medication dose. She soon looked drunken and tired. Quickly, this mistake caused commotion and great concern among the hospital staff.

- *Receiving medical treatment for a physical condition requires a different hospital with both medical and psychiatric support.* Due to an acquired bladder condition while at H2, paramedics transported me via ambulance to H3. A patrol car, with sirens blaring, entered the hospital emergency roundabout ahead of my ambulance. "The police are here to arrest me," I repeated to Rick. Of course, Rick knew there was never a factual basis for this outburst.

- *Illness and obedience don't always mesh.* The Social Worker at H3 had us patients jump in place for exercise. Though a catheter for my bladder infection was present, I still dutifully bounced up and down. An observing nurse seemed to purposely laugh at me, perhaps because I was foolish enough to bend and stretch with a catheter.

- *It appears even the hospital staff didn't like me.* Upon my recovery from the bladder infection, a nurse in H3 removed the catheter while I lay in my hospital bed. A small bit of urine soiled the top sheet. Neither she nor the other nurses offered new bedding. Later, when I asked for clean sheets, a male nurse handed me old, smelly, dank ones from the supply closet. "I guess I'm a problem patient who deserves these sheets," I thought. The truth is, I would have been better off keeping the original ones.

- *I often focused on an over-medicated patient at H1.* I remember a female patient that shuffled down the hall every day ever-so-slowly—sometimes with the aid of hospital personnel but most often on the arms of kindly patients within the facility. She spoke softly and repeatedly about how much she was a burden to her family. She mumbled this to herself, her fellow patients, her visiting husband, and her visiting daughters. Several weeks later, she and I met up at the H2 month-long outpatient facility. Now she was highly verbal, appearing sane, striding with an average gate, and no longer ruminating about being a problem to others. I spoke to her about the many kindnesses I noticed both staff and patients provided her at H1. She explained that others had verbalized to her precisely what I said, though she didn't remember much of it. With a degree of disdain, she also said that she was so overmedicated at H1 that she, indeed, was not herself. Hearing her scorn brought me a degree of comfort since I, too, felt over-medicated. Witnessing her change from zombie-like to normal was encouraging.

As a reader, you may see this list as the rantings of a dissatisfied hospital consumer. Or you may be horrified by my gruesome mindset. You might even find it quite unbelievable that hospital staff was selective in their treatment of different mentally ill patients. In my pre-hospital life, I had a reputation among friends, family, and employers as a genuinely kind, thoughtful woman. However, to those who met me during my hospitalization, I was deemed radically different.

Words are inadequate to explain the felt sense of internal and external chaos that surrounded me every moment of every day in all three hospitals for one solid month. Was it chaos? Was it psychosis? All of the above felt authentic to me. These events still appear to be "the facts as I remember them."

Gladly they no longer seem to matter much.

TAKEAWAYS

1. Though it was not my experience, some patients at H1 were helped by staff and were even grateful to be there. I know this because they told me so. I have seen other

family members supported by excellent therapy and treatment at their local psychiatric hospital. Take note that placement in a psychiatric hospital is a formidable option. In the end, though, it may be the only means of keeping you or your loved one safe.

2. If your loved one is in a psychiatric hospital, demand a list of what medications they are on. Read up on them and be able to describe to medical personnel any side effects.

3. Realize that pharmaceutical psychotropic drugs are powerful mind-shifters.

4. After being released from all three psychiatric hospitals, I truly benefitted from H2's month-long, six-hour-a-day outpatient clinic. My mom dropped me off every morning and picked me up each afternoon. The outpatient psychiatrist at H2-Outpatient Treatment was the first doctor to reduce my psychotropic medication doses. These decreases made a *huge* difference in changing, for the better, my personal experiences with chaos and psychosis. I am so grateful to him!

5. Losing weight, losing sleep, and losing the ability to read books due to a busy mind are all troublesome indicators

19

of depression or anxiety. The combination of all three is of great concern. Medical action (though it may not require hospitalization) is needed.

6. There's a sad, sideways synchronicity between the film, *What Dreams May Come*, and actor Robin Williams who played the struggling husband. Striving to pull his movie wife from her internal hell, in real life, Williams died by suicide in 2014. Sadly, the underlying cause of William's death was a rare brain disease called Lewy Body Dementia.[4]

7. Ten years from now, treating mental illness in hospital settings may catch up to some exciting alternatives happening now, including NeuroStar Advanced Therapy for Mental Health[5], Alpha-Stim[6], and Brain-Tap[7].

Chapter 3

SHAME

After my hospitalizations, admitting to others out loud that I was depressed and not fully functioning in this world took years to acknowledge. Of course, that small circle of family members and friends closest to me knew that I continued to struggle with depression. They still held deep concerns for me and wanted to be of help, yet we rarely discussed my depression. I could, however, commiserate with my sister, Julie, who had her own simultaneous struggles with depression and anxiety. "How did we *both* get here?" was often the question on our lips.

Writing this memoir, describing in detail what depression and anxiety felt like for me, still elicits some emotion. Yet, even so, I can talk about it openly with relative ease and have been able to do so since April 2015. That was the month I was asked to speak in my church on any subject of my choosing. As a depressed person, finding a topic was difficult for me when the only issue that resonated and seemed relevant was my current fight with depression. Simultaneously, I also suffered from what some call a severe "faith crisis." I had many doubts about specific teachings in my faith, which resulted in me leaving the church for seven years.

I ended up speaking about both things.

My willingness to share across the podium my struggles seemed to strike a chord within the congregation. So many expressed their compassion and goodwill when the meeting was over, and tender letters and emails followed. But my church family was not the only one affected by this experience. Talking publicly about my depression was the breakthrough that opened the door for me to feel less humiliation, loss of respect for myself, and fear of reproval from others. Apparently, some in the congregation experienced a similar breakthrough. From then on, the shame I felt around my mental illness lessened—and, best of all, eventually went away.

However, even with my most intimate therapists (Heather Braley, LMFT, and later DeBora Miller, LMFT—both of whom I deeply trusted), it felt as if I could state the facts but not open up genuinely to the more serious aspect of my depression. As I recall, they may have gently broached the subject. But for me, a deeply personal discussion was off-limits. In truth, I am a person who survived a suicide attempt.

You see, that October afternoon, following my discharge from Hospital 1, my mother took me to the local pharmacy to fill the several psychotropic medication prescriptions written by the H1 psychiatrist only hours before. We did not realize at the time how dangerous my access to those pills would be. Even still, the day before my release, both Rick and my mother begged that same doctor to keep me in the hospital. Both believed I was not ready to come home.

On my first morning back home, thoughts of Ophelia, the young woman gone mad in Shakespeare's play, *Hamlet*, came to mind. Queen Gertrude reported that Ophelia climbed into the branches of a willow tree. The limb holding Ophelia broke under her. She fell into the river below and drowned.

Then came other thoughts. "If one pill already makes my heart pound hard," I reasoned, "what would taking three pills do? Make it mercifully stop?" These voices in my head battled incessantly. "Take the pills." "Don't take the pills." "Take the pills." "Don't take the pills."

Although I wanted the extreme thoughts to go away, those mighty voices within me were reckless and impulsive.

Eventually, "Take the pills" won.

After taking two times more than the amount of Seroquel prescribed, I chose to lie in our backyard under the large oak tree, hoping my heart would pound hard enough to eventually stop beating. I don't think I lay there more than ten minutes before realizing death wasn't happening today. I hadn't taken enough. And it didn't cross my mind to take more.

I got up, weaving into the house and moving sloppily down the hall. While in a foggy haze, I dressed myself, then went out to the car for my first scheduled appointment at an outpatient clinic. Rick and my mom drove me to Hospital 2 for what we initially thought were outpatient services. However, once you overdose, you are on a different track.

It was only during my intake interview that Rick and my mother heard for the first time that I had not taken the prescribed 300 mg pill but instead had taken three pills—900 mg of Seroquel, before arriving. No, I didn't take the whole bottle. No, I didn't shove other prescription medications down my throat. No, I didn't scavenge for over-the-counter drugs in the medicine cabinet. In the medical world, taking more than what is prescribed is called an overdose—intention matters, and mine was to leave this planet.

My flirt with death changed who I was to hospital personnel. I was put on a gurney, placed in an ambulance, and sent to a standard hospital emergency room. After keeping me for evaluation, I was placed on another gurney, set in a different ambulance, and hurriedly deposited at the intake office of what would be the second psychiatric hospital I would attend—Hospital 2 (H2).

My attempt also changed how my husband and mother perceived me. Rick bought a heavy, black, Sentry fireproof safe with keys only he and my mom would possess. They supplied prescription medications specific to Jean Stoddard at the appropriate times and in the proper doses from their hands to mine.

It also changed how I perceived myself. Being treated like a child, I felt like a child—albeit a potentially dangerous one.

Taking two *extra* Seroquel became my most shameful deed.

Over the years, several people have expressed how selfish they believe a person is who chooses to die by suicide. As an attempt survivor, I don't honestly know how to respond to such a statement except to say, "It's not that simple."

Yes, one could judge my thinking as selfish; however, from my perspective, the mental anguish was unbearable. It felt as if depression would go on for the rest of my life. To think that I would live each coming day for years in agony made daily living intolerable. The pain in my brain was excruciating, and I wanted it gone. I even felt that God would understand.

Though it is now written here for all to see, my suicide attempt is not something I talk about with ease. I do so in the belief that by sharing my final remnants of shame with you, the disgrace I feel around it will lessen. I trust that honesty and openness have the power to dissolve shame, eventually making it disappear altogether.

TAKEAWAYS

1. Discussing depression revealed me to be a vulnerable, struggling human being. Those others who showed me, in return, a generous degree of compassion, empathy, and kindness weakened the hold shame had on me.

2. The admission of depression to trusted therapists, and later, most powerfully, to a larger group lessened my shame around it. Perhaps this admission of my suicide attempt will reduce my shame around that, too.

3. In my opinion, all good therapy gently moves you toward your pain and not away from it. Moving toward pain is doable with the right help but not easy work.

4. I believe that moving toward understanding the shame helps to release it, too.

5. There is better news. Doreen Marshall from the National Office of the American Foundation for Suicide Prevention (AFSP) states, "Someone who has made a suicide attempt has not put themselves in a category of permanent

fragileness." She concludes, "Mental illness is a health issue. Help is available."

6. I have devoted a chapter to helpful information and statistics from the AFSP.

7. There is a good chance you don't share my religion and may not share my spiritual beliefs. No worries. Our commonality will shine through if you can translate my spiritual language into yours. While reading my April 2015 church talk, perhaps focusing on the exquisiteness of what depression still felt like for me will be our common connection. (See Appendix A.)

Jean Conley Stoddard

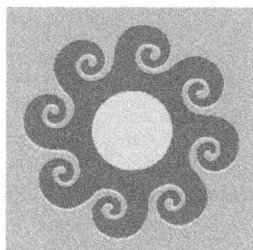

Chapter 4

THE IMPORTANCE OF EXCELLENT THERAPY

Upon returning home from the three hospitals, my new therapist, Heather, picked me up from my fall off the cliff. We worked together for one-and-a-half years. In part, a Jungian therapist, Heather chose instead to focus on relational therapy by helping me reengage with my family, church, and the world. The validation I received from Heather was highly comforting. She was an excellent talk therapist, and I felt safe with her and clearly understood.

Each week she would greet me from behind the white-painted door of her darling, therapeutic cottage among the pines. I relished drinking herbal tea made from her quick-heating warming pot.

Early on, she had Rick and my mom come in. She wanted their perspectives on my mental stressors. She invited me to remain in the room, hearing their views and reactions. Staying was not easy for me, though I believe it was helpful for both Rick and my mom. As for Heather, this raw insight helped her to help me.

Ten months after my hospitalizations, Rick was diagnosed with thyroid cancer. My mental state began to regress. Heather warned me that it was common for those with a mental illness to reenter a psychiatric hospital for a second time. I *feared* that for myself! During one session, I remember lying on Heather's couch, feeling like she was witnessing me more like an entity—the thing I was back in the hospitals, now with a fixed determination to take over. During that problematic session, Heather wouldn't buy what I said. She wouldn't buy into what I did—lying there on the couch (though she let me stay positioned that way). Heather would not feed into my folly. I noticed a part of me that was a silent witness—an objective observer of my regression on the couch. That spectator saw, too, Heather's therapeutic counseling efforts on my behalf. In only one session, Heather helped me climb out of the hole I was digging for myself. In fact, she went down there with me and brought me back to my senses. I am so grateful she steadied me. I never did return to any of the three mental hospitals.

I cried the day Heather gently announced that she would move to Southern California in four months. Orange County was an eight-hour drive away when traffic was good. It's metaphorically a state away, though a short plane ride away, and easily a bus or train ride away. Of course, none of that was reasonably possible in terms of continuing our therapy relationship. Though Orange County is a phone call away, that was not an option Heather seriously suggested for me.

She did as directed by her profession and provided me with the names of three therapists in the area that might be a good fit. Now, mind you, I was still depressed—perhaps a category two hurricane lessening in strength but still living in its spiral rainbands. The idea of me interviewing three therapists on my own was daunting. But I had enough capacity to know that I still needed help.

I first looked to my friends for their referrals. I even asked my psychiatrist, Dr. Goldman, whom he might suggest. Yet after a month of slowly slogging through this process, I finally contacted Heather's three recommendations.

I spoke to one therapist on the phone, corresponded to another by email, and even interviewed Goldman's suggested therapist in her office for thirty minutes. I ended up choosing DeBora—one of Heather's references. I set up the first consultation in DeBora's brightly painted, yellow-walled office.

During our initial interview in 2014, I internally rolled my eyes when DeBora spoke of her brand of therapy, a combination of talk therapy and "doing" therapy (my phrase, which elicited the big eye-roll). Talk therapy was awesome. ("It doesn't belong to me. It's moving through me." OR "We forget that we are spirit having a human experience." OR "Don't look side to side, just look ahead where you are going." –DeBora has beautiful wisdom.)

"Doing" therapy, however, brought up much resistance. Though not spoken aloud to DeBora, I thought to myself, "Are you crazy? I'm depressed! I can hardly get out of bed, and yet you want me to do stuff? Therapy things? Did you not hear the first time that I AM DEPRESSED? Depressed people can't do things! We're depressed!"

Nonetheless, little by little, my Psychotherapist, DeBora, had me do things.

For example, it took me a very long time to make space for the "doing" activity of sitting twenty minutes a day, both morning AND evening, in quiet solitude with no other agenda than to check in with myself. At the beginning of each therapy session, DeBora would ask how my week went. She would then slip in ever-so-gently the question, "Were you able to sit this week?" I would sheepishly answer, "No," or make up some weak excuse. She didn't pry any further during that session. The following week, she would ask about my week, including whether I had made time to sit quietly. Each week for many months, my answer remained, "No."

DeBora never made me feel guilty, nor would she chastise me for not sitting. Like clockwork, however, I could count on her continued asking. She clearly felt "sitting" would be a powerful therapeutic tool for me.

It took many months to actually set the alarm, wake up, walk to the living room couch, and sit quietly by myself for twenty minutes. Initially, I loathed it. My mind was busy, and noticing my steady, incessant, ruminating thoughts felt disturbing. Still, I set the alarm, got up, and went through the same daily routine.

Surprisingly, there came the day when sitting every morning became *one thing* from DeBora's psychotherapy tool kit that I genuinely wanted to do!

And guess what? After two months of morning sitting, I heard within me the silent witness, my objective observer. It gently whispered and gave me a simple idea to do something nice— deliver freshly squeezed juice—to a struggling friend. Acting on this impression made me feel good.

Maybe another week passed with nothing memorable in my brain to do for others. But later, I heard a clarifying voice within providing a bit of wisdom to something I was struggling over. Wow! Niceties for me? —what a concept!

The more I began to sit quietly, the more I started hearing from the better, healthier part of me. The worth in others was occasionally unveiled. The value within me was, too!

I began to look forward to my morning sitting. Eventually, I authentically could say to DeBora, "Yes, I was able to sit last week." I learned to love morning sitting.

Today I am a certified Mindfulness Meditation Practice Instructor through the University of Holistic Theology. I am witness to lives transformed by the ancient practice of meditation which initially started with my own healing.

Who knew that this *doing* therapy could turn into *being*?

Later, DeBora spoke of Louise Hay's book, *You Can Heal Your Life*, ironically one I already owned but did me no good sitting on the shelf. As you'll read in a coming chapter, "doing" affirmations means creating a combination of powerful phrases and then repeating them over and over for days, weeks, and months. Again, a lot of "doing."

DeBora spoke of juicing for my husband Rick's health because of his thyroid cancer. Juicing, as you will read in the chapter on nutrition, turned out to be a major turning point for me in my struggles with depression, though I'm sure it was helpful for Rick, too. Juicing also requires "doing." It means getting in a car and buying fresh fruits and vegetables at a grocery store. It means washing that produce. It means pulling out the juicer and assembling it. It means juicing what you washed, drinking it, and cleaning up the mess. That's a lot of "doing."

At DeBora's recommendation, I also joined Food Matters TV (FMTV) for its health documentaries. I filled out Tices logs; watched the *Fat, Sick and Nearly Dead* DVD; discovered Yogananda; investigated probiotics; treated myself to an occasional massage; learned the Float Back technique, Progressive Relaxation, and practices utilized from the Hakomi method. At a moment's notice, I could go to "Shalom"—a safe place she helped me create in my head. I listened to Belleruth Naparstek; learned the Three-Fold Breath technique; focused on Thought Stopping; and participated in what turned out to be a powerful modality for me— Eye Movement Desensitization and Reprocessing (EMDR). These are only a few of the many experiential offerings DeBora provided from her psychotherapy tool kit.

Some offerings I heard then quickly forgot—they never quite stuck. Others would become an irreplaceable part of my life.

The most important thing I learned from DeBora, and therapy in general, is that getting well is *work*. It's a *job*. Not my therapist's job, not my psychiatrist's job, not the medicine's job, not any book's job. Healing from depression is pedal-to-the-metal work! It's a lot of "doing." It was *my* job to do the work!

I don't know the therapeutic word for feeling "solid." Perhaps in therapy, it's called being "integrated." Near the end of my time in therapy, I told DeBora that in all my years of living, from the moment I was born until that very moment in time, I had never felt "solid" before. But now, I was dense, grounded, and capable in a fashion that felt permanent and would never leave me. "Solid" meant that when my life was hard, I could live through the blowing tea kettle, take it off the stove, and now make tea. "Solid" still describes my current internal sense of well-being.

I may have described my solidity to DeBora for several months before her hints and final proposal that I didn't need to come to therapy anymore. She said that she would always be available for any bump in the road in my future, but that for now, I was free to go, be on my own, and live life on my terms. I had, indeed, successfully slogged through the valley of the shadow of death. I had done enough work.

For me, excellent therapy was critical. Heather picked me up and steadied me onto solid ground. DeBora finished the job by helping make me solid. With their expertise and very goodwill, I emerged out the other side! I am so very grateful.

And yes, I did the work!

TAKEAWAYS

1. When looking for a psychotherapist, it was my experience that I was able to schedule a free, face-to-face interview with one for thirty minutes. From the office waiting room feel, to

the therapist's choice of décor, and most especially during your verbal exchange, you will get some sense of whether this therapist is a good match for you.

2. Trust between a therapist and client is critical. It's KEY!

3. I saw a different (and it turns out not as helpful) therapist for three years before the hospitalizations. I didn't entirely trust her and honestly didn't feel understood by her, but I kept going back for reasons I cannot articulate even today. Some would say she took me too far, too fast. Others, that she harmed me. All I can say is that even if you choose someone that you later don't like or mesh with, you can stop going to that therapist. TRUST YOURSELF! Then choose another. Do it sooner (which would have been best) rather than later (like I, unfortunately, did).

4. There are many forms of therapy, including group work. You WILL find the method that works for you because you found the therapist or group whose advice you value and whom you trust.

5. My therapist DeBora used with me, in part, experiential modalities such as Cognitive Behavioral Therapy (CBT), Hakomi Therapy, and Trauma-Focused Therapy, offering a striking palate of different "doing" activities. Remember,

37

though, that all you initially have to do is ONE thing! Choose the one that resonates. Make it your job. Do it until it's done.

6. Then guess what? Choose the next thing until you complete that one. In time, "doing" grows exponentially. It takes on a life of its own. The day will come when you can do much more than one thing!

7. Sitting, meditating, being still, whatever you want to call it, is a journey into your inner world. It's a powerful practice, but it came later when I'd done enough other work that the hurricane had lessened its grip considerably.

8. My hope for you is that you find the strength and ability to do the hard work of getting well—one "doing" thing at a time.

Chapter 5

THE IMPORTANCE OF GOOD PHARMACOLOGY

Pharmacology, a scientific medical term for drugs and, in my case, their therapeutic use, was a tough slog—at least in the beginning.

When I first set foot in Hospital 1 (H1), I took only one prescribed medication—Armour Thyroid 90 mg for hypothyroidism (low thyroid).

However, the H1 psychiatrist immediately prescribed for me Cephalexin 500 mg (an antibiotic); Seroquel 300 mg (a mood disorder drug); Sertraline HCL 100 mg (an anti-depressant—think Zoloft); and Bupropion HCL 10 mg (another anti-depressant—think Wellbutrin).

I found it difficult to believe that the drugs given to me in the hospital actually helped. I once overheard a conversation between Rick and the psychiatrist in which she said, "Jean is so small, and her body doesn't handle the medication well." What I needed most and craved deeply was sleep—I'd been without it for so long. I don't think any of the hospital medications helped me with insomnia. In fact, Seroquel, the mood disorder drug, made my heart race, thus, making sleep impossible.

My hospital-prescribed medications went with me to all three hospitals.

Unfortunately, upon my final release from these fortresses, I was left with the challenge of finding a psychiatrist who could monitor my progress and write pharmacological prescriptions for depression and anxiety. When finally home, I took the easy and financially feasible route of picking a psychiatrist nearby from an online list of several through our medical insurance policy. Though not very sympathetic, he quickly dropped my pill load down to one—the anti-depressant Wellbutrin. Wellbutrin helped me considerably for a while—until it eventually didn't.

In September 2012, still depressed and now sinking from Rick's cancer diagnosis, a friend highly recommended I see psychiatrist Dr. Ronald Goldman, MD. However, Goldman was not a listed provider, so my health insurance did not cover his $300.00 per hour fee. My husband weakly protested my change of allegiance and the incurring debt. Feeling desperate, I went anyway.

"The least amount of medication that does the most good" is Dr. Goldman's mantra. Initially, he had me take Aripiprazole (think

Abilify), or Asenapine (think Saphris), or Gabapentin (think Neurontin), or Clonazepam (think Klonopin). I tried several other psychotropics, anti-psychotics, mood stabilizers, anti-depressants, neurostimulants, and anti-anxiety medications. A psychiatrist has a sizeable pharmaceutical toolkit. Goldman even took over the prescription for Armour Thyroid.

His methods first included filling out a lengthy intake questionnaire and a five-page symptom checklist. The initial face-to-face interview was two hours long. After diagnosis, I checked in by phone shortly after he prescribed or tweaked a specific drug probing to know of its effectiveness. If that drug didn't work, he quickly switched it for another. He trusted me to perceive what was and was not working within my body.

Looking within to discern if a medication was working at first felt like a massively frightening responsibility. Perhaps you will remember that early on, Rick and my mom locked my depression meds into a safe because they didn't trust me to take the proper amounts. Goldman was now handing me the responsibility for discerning the efficacy of a drug on my mood. This scary task, however, turned out to be the very best thing. I began to trust myself.

Initially, Goldman and I met in his office bi-weekly. Over time we met monthly, then once every two or three months. The medications he originally tweaked began to work effectively. The better I felt, the more he began to cut back dosages. His adage, "The least amount of medication that does the most good," rang true! I started to feel more normal.

A couple of years passed before the day finally came when he removed me from all depression and anxiety medication. Hallelujah! Changing my diet through juicing and eating healthy food (putting many more fresh fruits and vegetables into my body) contributed in a huge way to getting me off pharmaceuticals for depression. I now was only on Armour Thyroid—ironically, the one medication I took when I first entered the mental hospital those years before. For me, getting off all depression and anxiety pills took four years with Dr. Goldman's careful monitoring. Thank you, Dr. Goldman!

The medication merry-go-round is a tough slog because, as founder Joshua Rosenthal from the Institute for Integrative Nutrition would say, we are "bio-individual" human beings. What works in one body may not work in another. The list of possible anti-depressant medications alone on the WebMD website numbers forty-seven in total—a number that will undoubtedly continue to grow.[1]

New drugs for depression, approved by The U.S. Food and Drug Administration (the FDA), come out all the time. Doctors—especially psychiatrists and pharmacists, must keep up with the new pharmacology.

In the medical community, taking medication appears to be the first initial step in treating depression. But it may take time to find the right one that works for you. Some conditions may become worse when the drug is stopped suddenly. So, the advice to not stop taking medication without consulting your doctor is solid.

For several years I was truly helped by taking psychotropic medication for depression. I did begin to feel better.

With the help of your doctor, I hope you find a medication that helps you. And may the day eventually come that you can live vibrantly without it!

TAKEAWAYS

1. As with a good therapist, liking and trusting your psychiatrist is essential.
2. In truth, prioritizing my mental health was a matter of life or death!

3. Health insurance may make shopping for a psychiatrist harder—not impossible, just a little trickier. Or you can pay on your own where the shopping is easier, though more expensive.

4. In the beginning, support from family or friends during your psychiatric appointments is worth considering. They may see things in your demeanor or behavior that you don't, thus providing a more comprehensive explanation of your conduct to the doctor.

5. Most pharmacies include a drug facts label and medication guide with your prescription regarding the drug's dosage, warnings and precautions, and adverse reactions. Read, or have your trusted family member or friend read that label and guide. Take the side effects warnings seriously! If you experience any of them, contact your doctor immediately!

6. Also, note that the FDA website has an alphabetized list of FDA-approved drugs. Check for your drug, and then click the "Medication Guide" link for all the facts.[2]

7. FYI hypo-thyroid symptoms may include depression.

8. In my experience, good nutrition played a significant role in helping me get off depression and anxiety medications.

Chapter 6

THE IMPORTANCE OF EXCEPTIONAL NUTRITION

In 2015, two-and-a-half years after Rick's thyroid cancer diagnosis, my therapist, DeBora, suggested juicing as a way to strengthen his immune system. I was still depressed though improving; I was still panicked that Rick would die; and I still felt certain I could not do life independently without his help. DeBora shared her own juicing success story with me and mentioned something about an Australian guy (Joe Cross) who juiced his way across America while losing weight. His story is in the documentary *"Fat, Sick and Nearly Dead."*

I watched the film, now convinced juicing would help Rick.

I am not talking about making and drinking freshly squeezed orange juice. No, I am talking about medicinal juicing with, for example, a half piece of fruit followed by carrots, tomatoes, spinach, and kale.

I told Rick that DeBora suggested juicing for his health and offered to make it for him daily. However, it was no surprise to me that he abruptly said, "No."

The only chance I had for Rick to possibly drink this kind of juice was to try out medicinal juicing for myself. I purchased a Joe Cross book explaining why and how to juice. It included several recipes. "Perhaps," I thought, "I could offer tastes to Rick." I wished that someday he would drink them by simply watching me.

Next, I pulled out my twelve-year-old, trusty Champion Juicer—the one I brought out every winter to juice the local Satsuma mandarins purchased in twenty-five-pound lug crates from our local Placer County orchards.

To my amazement, after four days of juicing for myself, I started feeling more energetic. I got up early to make fresh juice. I started vacuuming the living room carpet. I showered!

Rick noticed.

Soon he told me he would drink the juice I made. I doubled the recipe and gave him eight ounces of juice daily—simply one-measured cup!

However, Rick would gag, complain about the taste, or make these weird grimaces while grunting his disapproval. It annoyed me a lot! I had to leave the room at the first sound of his displeasure.

Eventually, I took the hint and stopped making juice for him altogether. A couple of days passed until one morning, however, he asked, "Where's my juice?" "Seems to me you don't like it," I cynically replied, "so I stopped making it." Though he didn't disagree, he said he still wanted to drink the juice.

I was as ecstatic as a depressed person could be but kept a stoic face. ("Maybe Rick won't die this year, after all!" I thought.)

Several months later, Rick went to his general practitioner physician to get his regular six-month checkup which always included blood work. After the appointment, he told me that the doctor had asked him what new activities he had been doing because his lab numbers had changed positively, and he was no longer pre-diabetic. Also, the doctor now planned to cut his cholesterol medication in half. Rick told him the only thing he could think of that changed was drinking a cup of freshly squeezed "medicinal" vegetable juice every day.

I was again as thrilled as a depressed person could be from the doctor's report—a confirmation that maybe Rick won't die this year, after all! (And by the way, Rick is still alive at the printing of this book!)

At the same time, Dr. Goldman was slowly weaning me away from the various depression medications he and others before him had prescribed. However, when juicing came on the scene, getting off psychotropic medications sped along with great intensity.

In 2016, I became a Dr. Goldman success story. I am totally off all psychotropic prescription medications. Yes, I genuinely am grateful to my excellent Psychiatrist and all he did initially using psychiatric drugs to help me during the rough patch. But I also feel I owe much to medicinal juicing. Juicing gave me increased energy and, as my husband puts it, "increased capacity." My cells became Pac-Man-like, gobbling up the vitality they received from authentic nutrition.

Juicing has evolved, with celery juicing becoming the newest vegetable drink phenomenon. Both Rick and I drink 8 ounces per day.

Juicing began my significant health journey in which I:

- took a nutrition class at the local community college.
- explored a vegan diet through the Physicians Committee for Responsible Medicine's 21-day Kick Start program.[1]
- joined the Forks Over Knives vegan cooking school.
- graduated from the Institute for Integrative Nutrition's health coach training program.

One step led to a healthier other.

Remember that these NATURAL, POWERFUL, and BEAUTIFUL fruits and vegetables are medicine to your body and mind. Eat them generously!

Recollect that as "bio-individual" human beings, what works for one may not work for another. Experiment to determine what works for you!

Health means everything.

TAKEAWAYS

I have had plenty of doctors, dieticians, and nutritionists tell me that they don't like juicing because it affects people's blood sugar levels and that fiber (important in scrubbing the large intestines and helping with elimination) is removed during juicing. Yes, they make a good case. However, Rick and I drink only one cup of fresh, organic vegetable juice daily. That means we currently drink more celery in one juice than we would have been able to eat in one sitting. I don't know if juicing is for you. It was a compelling option, however, for my healing from depression.

Here are some considerations:

- Juicers mainly come in two types—centrifugal and masticating.

- Centrifugal juicers are cheaper, but their motors are less powerful. They leave more juice in the pulp, though you can put the pulp in an almond milk bag, squeezing it firmly to get out the remaining liquid.

- I prefer masticating juicers. Masticating juicers are more expensive because they have more powerful motors. They squeeze more juice out of the pulp. The Champion brand noted above is a masticating juicer. I later purchased an Omega 8006. In my opinion, there is no perfect juicer, and juicers still are amazing.

- One option is to borrow or buy a USED juicer before taking the juicing plunge. Juicing is an investment of both time and money. Juicing also involves a lot of clean-up. It's a bit of a learning curve! In the beginning, perhaps a loved one will put in the time to make juice for you.

- You can freeze juices though the Medical Medium author and celery juice proponent, Anthony William, says not to freeze celery juice.

- Joe Cross has something to say about juicing's benefits. Check out his Reboot with Joe website.[2]

Regarding nutrition:

1. I don't necessarily love the taste of celery juice. My feelings in that regard are neutral. Rick, on the other hand, dutifully and willingly drinks his glass every day but always refers to it as "the nasty," even if I'm not there to hear it.

2. In my Western culture, I believe that most people don't eat enough fresh fruits or vegetables. All you need to do is start with just one thing! Trust yourself to start putting one more vegetable on your plate or in your glass.

3. The Environmental Working Group's Guide to Pesticides in Produce distributes its *Clean 15* and *Dirty Dozen* list annually. The *Clean 15* list shows edible produce with little worry of pesticide contamination. *The Dirty Dozen* list is concerning.[3]

4. "Product ingredients are listed (on food labels) by quantity—from highest to lowest amount; therefore, the first ingredient is what the manufacturer used the most of."[4]

5. There's a fascinating story of Kathleen DiChiara, who claimed health for herself and her medically suffering family, in the documentary *Secret Ingredients*.[5] This movie speaks to eliminating genetically modified food (GMOs) from your diet and eating organically. DiChiara has since

become a Functional Diagnostic Nutrition Practitioner with several other certifications.

6. If you eat meat, eggs, or fish, then grass-fed, antibiotic-free, hormone-free, and wild are important considerations.

7. In the past, eating sugar in all its varieties was a problem for me. My former therapist Heather has this to say about sugar. "Sugar is a highly addictive, white, crystalline substance, and Americans are practically snorting it." She believes the day will come when warning labels on sugary food packages will be the norm, similar to those now on cigarettes.

8. If you start feeling well through better nutrition, discuss with your psychiatrist your desire to be slowly and carefully weaned off your medications but ONLY WITH THE DOCTOR'S SUPERVISION!

Chapter 7

THE POWER OF POSITIVE AFFIRMATIONS

One of the cognitive-behavioral treasures in my former therapist DeBora's experiential therapy toolkit is the book she challenged me to read, *You Can Heal Your Life*, by Louise Hay. Ironically, it's one I owned and glanced at but had never put into practice. Now, willing to reconsider the book and possibly do one thing from it, I chose from the list of "problems" at the back. Those particular to me included anxiety, depression, and suicide.

I compiled an affirmation from her "new thought pattern" list that goes like this:

I LOVE AND APPROVE OF MYSELF. I LIVE IN THE TOTALITY OF POSSIBILITY. THERE IS ALWAYS ANOTHER WAY. I AM SAFE. I NOW GO BEYOND ANY FEARS AND LIMITATIONS. I CREATE A NEW LIFE WITH NEW RULES THAT TOTALLY SUPPORT ME. I AM WILLING TO CHANGE.

Concentration to learn this affirmation was hard-won. My depression was dark and heavy-laden, while the anxiety made my mind spin too fast to focus. So, I typed the affirmation out on the computer, taped a large print copy on my car dashboard, and kept a duplicate in my wallet. I repeated those seven sentences over, and over, and over, and over. Finally, after two weeks, I memorized them all. Then came the actual work. I repeated the entire affirmation for minutes, days, weeks, and yes, even months while the other voice in my head still shouted its opposing message.

Repeating affirmations might feel pointless to you or seem too simplistic. It's not.

These two voices—the depressed one and the affirming one— competed for my psyche. The depressed voice yelled loudest and strongest. After all, it had kept me unwelcome company for several years. I believed those heavy, negative thoughts were me, that they were true, and that they would be with me for the rest of my life.

Initially, the new affirming voice was outside of me. I spoke my affirmation by rote, paper in hand, as if I were shoving the words against my temples with a clenched fist while seeking for any opening to push them through. The affirmation did not feel true for me. "I am safe?" "I live in the totality of possibility?" "I mean, who says that to themselves?" I thought.

About three months in, without ever truly believing anything would change significantly, I woke one morning noticing something subtle and new. My eyes looked around, questioning. "What's going on? What is this? Something's different. What's changed?" I asked. "Oh, wow............ it's *hope*! I haven't felt hope in *years*! Where did that come from?" I wondered. "Your affirmation, Jean!" replied my inner knowing.

Hope came. And hope stayed!

Louise Hay teaches, *"Learn to think in positive affirmations. Affirmations can be any statement you make. Too often, we think in negative affirmations. Negative affirmations only create more of what you say you don't want. Saying, 'I hate my job,' will get you nowhere. Declaring, 'I now accept a wonderful new job,' will open the channels in your consciousness to create that."*

Hay adds, "Continually make positive statements about how you want your life to be. However, there is one point that is very important in this: *Always make your statement in the PRESENT TENSE*, such as 'I am' or 'I have.' Your subconscious mind is such an obedient servant that if you declare in the future tense, 'I want,' or 'I will have,' then that is where that idea will always stay—just out of your reach in the future!" (Louise Hay, *You Can Heal Your Life*, 76)

Affirmations are powerful. Language is powerful. Words are powerful. What we say to ourselves—our inner conversation—can take us down or build us up. Repeatedly saying my POSITIVE affirmation was one of the most important things I did to heal from depression. *I cannot emphasize enough how powerful and transformative doing this was!*

My hope for you is that internalized hope will come to you. And that hope will stay. Perhaps repeatedly stating your positive affirmation is the one thing you can do right now.

TAKEAWAYS

1. Create a positive affirmation.
2. Make a copy of your affirmation for your car and tape it to the dashboard. Put a copy in your purse or wallet. Trust that the day will soon come when you will have it memorized.
3. You won't believe the affirmation at first. I didn't believe it. Say it anyway! Say it hundreds of times a day for weeks and even for months. You can affect your thinking more positively with this continual effort!
4. Louise Hay suggests saying your affirmation to yourself while looking in a mirror. I did not do it that way, but she implies that affirmations work faster by adding mirror work.

5. If I had an fMRI taken of my brain before saying my affirmation and a scan after hope came, I believe that comparing the two fMRIs would show a definitive change. We can re-wire our brains. Adults, not just the youthful, can grow new telomeres at the ends of their chromosomes. We can grow new neural networks. It is my experience that stating positive affirmations is one of the ways.

6. I hope for you that in stating your positive affirmations repeatedly, you will eventually find relief for your troubled, tired brain and a new lens through which to see your improved world.

7. *Positive affirmations are powerful!* I still have mine memorized to draw upon occasionally, should I need it.

8. Affirmations are trusted friends.

Jean Conley Stoddard

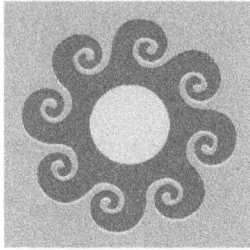

Chapter 8

MEDITATION IS ANCIENT THERAPY

"So," you ask, "How does a person who spent one month in three different mental hospitals, slogged four more years through pretty serious depression, and, by the way, it's hard to forget you went to hell and back, become a Mindfulness Meditation Instructor?"

I dabbled in yoga during high school. I read Jon Kabat-Zinn's *Full Catastrophe Living* in the '90s. And as you learned earlier, my therapist DeBora took the idea of *sitting still* out of her therapy toolkit. *Sitting still* is the gentler term for the more transcendent one—meditation. This regularity of sitting is called a "practice."

Concentration is the first of three significant minds that show up in mindfulness meditation practice. Meditators initially learn to anchor at their breath because, face it, the breath happens in the present moment. It's as if "we are being breathed," states author Byron Katie in her book, *Loving What Is*. However, severely depressed people CAN'T concentrate. When I left my husband at the end of the college spring semester, I received A's in my two

59

college accounting classes. However, four months later, I found the next semester's class—managerial accounting—impossible to finish. My mind ruminated endlessly over all the things I felt paralyzed in attempting. Within seconds my brain hurled back and forth, doubting every decision. It's a miracle that I withdrew from that class without penalty.

Mindfulness is the most significant and vital brain characteristic in meditation. It includes the kind, thoughtful, aware, peaceful, and loving parts within each of us. One must be quiet to hear our better part share its gentle wisdom. In meditation circles, this regularity of sitting still is called a "practice."

Saddled with depression, however, the mind I was listening to was neither concentrative nor mindful. It was, instead, the third mind known in meditation as *the ego*. My brain was the "shrieking, gibbering madhouse on wheels barreling pell-mell down the hill, utterly out of control and helpless," labeled by Bhante Gunaratana in his book, *Mindfulness in Plain English*. And his description is for those who aren't necessarily depressed!

Kudos, of course, go back over 2500 years to Prince Siddhartha Gautama, later honored with the title Buddha or "enlightened" one. During the last forty-five years of the Buddha's life, he generously taught "only suffering and the transformation of suffering" to anyone who would listen. He was pointing to the way out of our suffering minds.

The Buddha himself shifted from egoic thinking to mindful thinking, and we can, too. Recently deceased Zen Buddhist monk Thich Nhat Hanh calls the ego "the storm-of-the-mind." He assured us that, "We can put an end to our suffering just by realizing that our suffering is not worth suffering for." (*The Heart of the Buddha's Teaching: Transforming Suffering into Peace, Joy, and Liberation.*)

I became a certified Mindfulness Meditation Instructor through the University of Holistic Theology in May 2019.

TAKEAWAYS

1. I don't know if your tsunami has passed or if you still live with a Category 5 hurricane. Start as DeBora suggested and sit quietly with your eyes closed for a brief, daily, designated time. If you can't do 20 minutes at first, try five minutes (or less). Even if you don't like doing it today, try it tomorrow.

2. Your mind will wander. It does for everyone! Scientists even have a name for it—the "default mode network." And yes, with depression, it roams obsessively. Over time, however, you will begin again to hear your more mindful self. It takes

time to notice any differences or positive changes in all healing practices.

3. Be mindful of whether you are a morning person or a night owl. Schedule your sitting accordingly.

4. Since I am guessing you don't sleep very well, you may have the good fortune of falling asleep during some of your sitting times. That's OK initially, but in truth, Mindfulness Medication Practice is active.

5. *The Mindful Vegan: A 30-Day Plan for Finding Health, Balance, Peace and Happiness* by Lani Muelrath is the best beginner's Mindfulness Meditation Practice book I have come across because it combines meditation education with guided meditation. Within 30 days of applying its principles, you will have created an authentic meditation practice.

6. If you want to learn more about meditation, I have several Mindfulness Meditation Practice videos on YouTube. Simply type my name in the YouTube search bar—Jean Stoddard.

7. The mind that is depressed and anxious is one manifestation of the *egoic* mind. When depressed, the ego's powerful voice is all you hear. Would you agree that the egoic mind is exhausting?

8. No one describes the egoic and mindful minds better than Eckhart Tolle. His book, *The Power of Now*, is the most beautifully written dictionary of both minds. He uses hundreds of words to point to the *ego* and the word he prefers for mindfulness is *presence*.

9. To begin meditation, you close your eyes. With less distraction and no looking about, shutting your eyes helps you go inward.

10. Next, you follow the acronym PAIR, coined in Muelrath's book, previously noted. PAIR stands for position, anchor, intention, and remindfulness.

11. POSITION, in the United States, involves sitting in a chair. Set yourself up for success and comfort. Hands go on thighs or stay cupped in your lap.

12. ANCHOR is what holds your concentration—initially at the breath and later at the body and emotions. You can choose one breath anchor among many options, for example, the nostril tips, the sinuses, the chest, the abdomen, or the pauses at each end of the breath.

13. INTENTION always includes a time frame. Ten minutes a day is powerful and comes with a promise. "By sitting and mindfully breathing for ten minutes a day, in as little as eight

weeks you strengthen the part of the prefrontal cortex involved in generating positive feelings and diminish the part that generates negative ones." (Richard Davidson, PH.D. *10 Mindful Minutes* by Goldie Hawn and Wendy Holden, 61).

14. REMINDFULNESS is the process of meditation itself. The concentrative, egoic, and mindful minds are always present during meditation. You a) concentrate on the breath, b) the egoic mind travels, and c) the mindful mind notices and brings you back to concentration. Like using a fishing pole, it reels you back. It reminds you to return to primary anchor at the breath—remindfulness! It's cyclical and very much like a waltz—one, two, three, one, two three.

15. As a beginner, it's critical to understand that effective meditation is not at first about stilling your mind. Initially, it is simply about noticing that the egoic mind has drifted one of two places—to a future that hasn't happened yet or to the past. We all do it. It's normal. Our thinking "defaults" when we are not concentrating.

16. When you later learn to anchor at your body and emotions through various body scanning techniques, you come to understand why Mindfulness Meditation Practice is *ancient*

therapy! Your body knows what hurts on a cellular, physiological level through its innate awareness of respiration and sensations. Pay enough attention, and eventually, your mind will know, too.

17. Meditation could be your "one thing."

18. DeBora reminded me, however, that "Some people are unable to sit still or close their eyes or be quiet. It is too activating for them. It would be too big an ask for them to sit alone quietly. It could trigger a panic attack. Every person is different and has different capabilities based upon their history and biological makeup. Ultimately, a therapist may want to help a person get to a mindfulness practice, but it may not be as simple as it was with you, Jean."

19. If it is too soon to be your "one thing," that's okay, too.

Jean Conley Stoddard

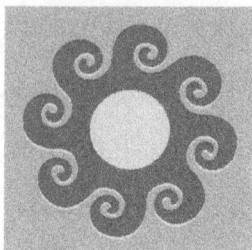

Chapter 9

SUPPORT LOOKS LIKE THIS

My mom flew from her home in Gulfport, Florida, to mine near Sacramento, California, within days of my entering Hospital 1 (H1). She bought a one-way ticket, not knowing when she would return to Florida but with a willingness to stay as long as she was needed. Initially, I didn't want my mom to come cross country because I didn't intend for her to see me this way.

She came anyway.

Who needed her? Most assuredly, Rick, now with a mentally disabled wife to whom he quickly realized, could not be left alone in the house. He would benefit from a pair of listening ears to bounce around ideas for my support. My mom being there enabled him to go peacefully off to work.

I didn't yet know that I needed Mom until she came with Rick every single day during all hospital visiting hours. She brought with her a small pile of clean clothes. She offered gentle hands that, at times, would take mine into hers. Her fixed determination was present for all the ugly and frightening.

After the hospitalizations, I didn't have the energy or wits to figure out what to eat. Feeding myself one meal a day, let alone three felt overwhelming. My mom cooked for me.

The dark voice in my brain was so loud and exhausting that my mom helped distract it by buying a flat-screen television and comfort movies to go with it. Romantic comedies, which caused me to smile for occasional, brief moments of relief, made welcome distracting sounds over my own dark voices. As I sprawled longways on the couch, Mom quietly kept me company in a neighboring chair.

She tried her best to understand why sometimes the bedroom carpet was the better place to sleep as I rolled up into a ball or rested my forehead hard on the floor in some effort to keep the dark voices at bay.

She loved the Dollar Tree stores and would make an outing of finding some $1.00 treasure that would give me or someone she cared about joy, even if it meant spending more in postage to send off her gem.

She traveled with Rick and me to our family in Tennessee during Thanksgiving when I couldn't find any energy to book the flights. (Rick did). I truly feared that I couldn't get on an airplane.

(Rick and Mom sat on either side of me). I felt certain there would not be enough of me available to converse and interact with my daughter, son-in-law, and five grandchildren, though the surprise was, I could.

Mom is the one who suggested I go back to "my" church, not "hers," which advice I eventually took her up on.

She stayed with Rick and me for three long, healing months. Then, ten months later, when Rick got his thyroid cancer diagnosis, she came out again for a month because I could feel I was spiraling downward again with the blow from his diagnosis.

My mother died in 2015. I love and miss her. If you could witness the tears falling from my eyes as I write this, you would know that my mother was there for me in every way possible during this crisis. She never got to see me at my very best in this life. She never saw me rise to become "solid." Though she saw me in my most weak and vulnerable state, I'll never forget how she carried me. I hope you can understand how very, very grateful I am for her. My hope for you is that you have, to some degree, that kind of support.

I hinted at "another perceived financial stress" in the introduction of this memoir. A second bankruptcy never materialized. And as you know, Rick took me back. He was there for me every day of my time in the three hospitals. He's never penalized me for leaving. What I have always valued in our relationship is that Rick has always let me be me. That didn't change with me leaving or in my becoming mentally ill. Our life together hasn't been easy. That's another story. However, Rick has always been kind. And I know he loves me. Thank you, Stodd. I love you.

My daughter Emily was Rick's go-between to get messages to other family members regarding my well-being and his. Sons and daughters telephoned me, but my memory of those hospital calls is hazy. You can read my son Allen's and daughter Mandy's experiences calling me during my stay in Hospital 1 in the chapter, *Reports from the Front Line.*

I am grateful to Rick's former employer, who gave me a low-stress job while I was still recovering from depression because he learned that Rick couldn't leave me home alone. This generosity allowed Rick to keep an eye on me at the company where we then both worked.

Friends wanted to reach out to me during my hospitalizations, but I avoided those conversations. My voice sounded dull, and my brain wasn't working. "What could we possibly talk about?" I thought. I was ashamed of my status as a depressed person going from mental hospital to mental hospital for thirty days. How could I ever begin to explain it to others? I didn't understand it myself.

Still, my friend Jan kept doggedly calling. When finally home, I eventually succumbed to her push toward connecting. She became the middleman friend I was willing to discuss my hurts with. She informed others of my status. Her words to me were always calm and reassuring. I never felt judged by her. She even made me laugh, which doesn't seem possible with depression. Jan didn't give up on me. How do I know that? By her actions—her relentless phone calls.

After leaving Rick, Dawn gave me a home while showing full concern. My friend Julie always gave me respite and goodwill pre and post-hospital stays. Alison later gave me a different job knowing my depression still wasn't gone. Tertia saw me raw and wounded and let me volunteer (whenever it suited me—not her) so that I could have the blessed distraction of working for a greater cause. Sabrina was my telephone lifeline before my hospitalizations and became the same for my mother during and after I came home. Kim supported me as I quickly spiraled downward and supported Rick in getting me to the hospital. As a counseling graduate, she saw what was happening through her therapeutic eyes.

Of course, my brother Tom supported me by supporting our mother. He took over her finances, check writing, and bill paying for the three months she was gone. My sister Julie commiserated with frequent check-ins by phone and email.

71

As you've read in other chapters, it goes without saying that my fabulous therapists—Heather and DeBora, as well as my exceptional psychiatrist, Dr. Goldman, supported me with excellent therapeutic and medical support.

When I said "OK" to going to the "dark side" the first night at Hospital 1, I didn't have a set belief system in place. I had been raised Catholic, changed religions at the age of twenty-three, married Rick in the "Mormon" temple in 1983, and left that church in 2004 with doubts and questions. However, this newly revealed "dark side" terrified me as it followed me to every hospital. Rick had offered to give me a priesthood blessing in H1, and I remember saying, "It's too late for that," believing I'd crossed over into a world from which I could not return.

Months later, when my mother suggested I return to "my church," I asked myself, "What is the opposite of what I experienced in the hospital?" And the response, "Jesus Christ." Then the question, "Where did I learn the most about the loving, kind Jesus?" The answer, "The LDS Church." Yes, I went back to my membership in The Church of Jesus Christ of Latter-Day Saints—still with my old questions and doubts, but now they didn't matter as much.

Here's what support from my church congregation leader at that time, Bishop Latham, entailed. He reassured me that I was a good person; that I had NOT crossed over to a world from which I could not return. At my request, we met weekly for many months. I received priesthood blessings from him and absorbed his gentlest and kindest counsel. When both therapist Heather and Bishop Latham suggested I find comforting scriptures and put them in a notebook, they heard my fear that because of depression, the scriptures were hard for me to read. The harsher messages within those pages re-wounded me. Bishop Latham generously looked for comforting scriptures but soon recognized that what I described made sense—consoling scriptures are harder to find. "But," he promised, "they are there." I now have two small notebooks full of the most reassuring scriptures I heard from the pulpit or read in a book. They continue to bless my life. Thank you, Bishop Latham, for being there when I was hurting so deeply from my fears.

To all who supported me during those tough, terrifying years, I love you so much. I am eternally grateful for everything you did for me. Support looks like YOU!

TAKEAWAYS

1. Remember that you have many friends and family that love you and would do anything to support you.

2. Remember, thoughts are powerful. Your thinking mind can take you down to the depths of hell or raise you to lofty heights. Guard your thinking.

3. In my notebook, the first three scriptures are Matthew 11:28 "Come unto me. All ye that labor and are heavy laden, and I will give you rest." D&C 50:16 "I will be merciful unto you; he (she) that is weak among you hereafter shall be made strong." Psalm 56:4 "In God I will praise his word; in God I have put my trust."

4. Positive scriptures read like affirmations. You can transform your favorite scriptures into positive sayings using "I" statements. Using Philippians 4:8 as an example: "Finally brethren (and sisters—Jean), whatsoever things *are* true, whatsoever things *are* honest, whatsoever things *are* just, whatsoever things *are* pure, whatsoever things *are* lovely, whatsoever things *are* of good report; if *there be* any praise, (I) think on these things."

5. Wise sayings became welcome additions to my notebook. They include words from other spiritual teachers like Louise Hay, Thich Nhat Hanh, Eckhart Tolle, Byron Katie, and Michael Singer, to name a few.

Chapter 10

REPORTS FROM THE FRONT LINE

May these reports from trusted friends and family living on the front line with loved ones and others who have suffered or still suffer from depression offer you sympathy, awareness, consolation, insight, and empathy. Their reports follow in the order received:

<u>"MERRY-GO-ROUND"</u> — Rick, Jean's husband

"This is a bad place," I thought after Jean's admittance to the first lock-down mental institution. *"This truly is the dark side."* At the same time, I was glad for her hospitalization because I felt she was safe from making a suicide attempt. Our daughter, with children who also had mental health issues, gave me some great advice. "Dad, don't get on the merry-go-round." "What does that mean?" I asked. "You will know when you get on and realize you have made a mistake," she cautioned.

I did not picture a traditional merry-go-round with colorful up-and-down horses but instead a playground spinner that twirls rapidly in tight circles making riders dizzy and disoriented. This whirling image helped me discern when I had erred and "got on."

Over time and even today, when advising others, I explain more succinctly that separate from staying off the merry-go-round, you need to be present, engaged, accepting, empathetic, and non-dismissive toward your mentally suffering loved one. But you can't "get on" with them when their reality is warped or otherwise not *the truth* of the situation, even to show support. The difference is a fine line, learned fully only by trial and error. You learn to pick and choose your battles.

In Hospital 1, when Jean told me that she wanted to kill our infant granddaughter, I just listened, with no specific response. I saw nothing to be gained by arguing that I felt she did not mean it. Conversely, I rebutted her worldview when Jean also told me that I should not revisit her because she was bad for me and would be arrested and put into prison later that evening. I explained how her thinking was not true, that she was *not* bad for me, and that her arrest and imprisonment would not happen. I would prove it tomorrow when we both saw that she was still in the hospital at the next visit.

Jean stopped telling me she was going to prison. Maybe I helped, or perhaps she continued to believe that way but chose not to share it with me—who can know for sure? All I could do for certain was visit her every time I was allowed—at *selective* moments challenging her thinking, but at *every* moment being as present and supportive as I could without getting on the merry-go-round.

"SPENCER CHRISTIAN, DEVOTED SON" — Name Withheld 1

My beloved son, Spencer, spent the last twelve years of his life fighting drug addiction. Concurrently, I was fighting *for* his life while feeling despair, desperation, at times an upswing of repeated hope, followed by the crash of witnessing another dreaded relapse. I hope very few of you will ever know this kind of emotional roller coaster.

My son loved to *play*—from guitar to sports like canoeing, baseball, and football. He was hardwired from birth to eat, sleep, and breathe athletics. He read sports statistics the way other kids read comic books. During junior high, he hit a baseball 425 feet, slamming it over the Simons Park Fence. Spence blocked a bigger boy during his freshman football season and pushed him all the way down the field. In the end, however, the football train containing Spencer's dream of playing college or pro ball had long left the station.

Things began cycling downward as Spencer turned sixteen. His stint in rehab offered no positive outcome. I pulled him out of high school at the end of his junior year to distance him from the surrounding atmosphere of drugs. The next day I took him to take the GED, in which he scored in the top 90 percentile. Then he took the Air Force Qualifying Test scoring a 93. However, Spencer had to lose weight to join the military, so four days later, he went to live with his sister, Sara, who was in the Air Force. Spencer proved to be a handful for her, and soon he returned home, only to experience the loss of his best friend to a heroin overdose. Spence then moved to New Orleans to help with restoration and clean-up after Hurricane Katrina. Spencer loved what he was doing in Louisiana. Best of all, he was clean!

That was until he came home again, and he wasn't.

Heroin is truly cunning—a powerful mind-controlling drug. I cannot count how many times Spencer would work through recovery only to relapse and then experience anger and self-loathing. I tried to help him understand that recovery is not about a bad person becoming good but rather about a sick person becoming well. But unfortunately, the lack of effective medical support made the cycle continue.

I gave Spence a book called, *Tweak: Growing Up on Methamphetamines*, a memoir by author Nic Sheff about his own battle with addiction using pot, cocaine, ecstasy, crystal meth, and heroin. Sheff felt he would always be able to quit and pull his life together whenever he needed to, and eventually, he did. After finishing the book, Spencer hugged me, kissed my cheek, and stated, "I could have written this book." Though Nic Sheff beat his addiction and lived, my Spencer was not able to "pull his life together when he needed to." He died on February 1, 2015.

Spencer had a brain disease—not a physical illness. An illness is something that resolves itself with temporary medication or treatment—like a cold or flu. Diseases like diabetes or high blood pressure, however, are not often resolved without continuous medication, treatment, or therapy. If you take away the medicine or treatment, the condition persists and often gets worse. Addiction is a disease—and in my son's case, it resulted in his untimely death at age twenty-eight.

When Spencer would play the Jackson Browne song "These Days" and heard the verse, "Don't confront me with my failures / I had not forgotten them," he would tap my arm and say, "Yes, I am guilty of that." None of us want to be known for our failures. Certainly, Spencer didn't want that. Instead, I would ask that an honest and transparent conversation surrounding drug addiction happens rather than simply "swiping up" our pain. Our communities need to become a lighthouse for families navigating this costly narco-terrorism destroying our cities.

Spencer Christian, I am so grateful that you are my son and so thankful to be your mom. I know your love for your family and me spurred on your continuous struggle to be clean. I respect, love, and honor you for that. My heart will always ache that your daughter will never know your laughter or love. If given the opportunity, we will share all that you were to us with her.

You will always be my loving, big-hearted, world's greatest hugger, and devoted son. I wait on the day when we will be together, and I will hear you say, "Hey Mom, where is the meatloaf?" and "What, no German Chocolate cake?" For now, I will forever celebrate your birth.

Happy Birthday, Spence.

SPENCER'S MOM organized his 2015 memorial service several months later, on October 11—Spencer's birthday.

"OUR BELOVED MOLLY" — Becky and Steve
Jean's longtime friends

Molly, the youngest of our five children, was 36 years old when she took her own life while alone in her apartment. Although six painful years have passed without her, writing this has still been very hard, though unexpectedly therapeutic.

Part of our sadness has been that so many people didn't get to know Molly or appreciate the incredible talents she used during her long periods of accomplishment and joy. She was a triumphant sprinter, relay athlete, and an excellent all-around student during junior high school. As a gifted seamstress, Molly blessed many with her beautiful quilts. Having learned how to bake from her grandparents, she treated countless family, friends, and even strangers to her delicious pastries. Molly was her mother's best friend, traveling companion, interior designer, and all-around helper.

Molly's death came after a long and courageous struggle with emotional challenges and mental illness. Since the age of sixteen, Molly had attempted suicide five times, miraculously surviving some of her more severe attempts. However, during the last four months of her life, she had distanced herself from us, not providing her telephone number or a way to contact her. We were devastated but not wholly surprised when we found out about her passing. To know she is permanently gone from us in this life is crushing. We miss her every day.

Steve and I loved Molly beyond measure and gave her everything we had to provide the love, security, and medical help that she needed. She suffered daily under significant burdens, which we found out much later, were brought about by severe abuse during her childhood. A secret cult in our neighborhood had done the unthinkable, subjecting Molly to forceful brainwashing and ongoing ritualistic sexual abuse. Molly hid the depth of her battles with this inner chaos—battles that medicine and counselors could not seem to soothe adequately. In the end, we believe that it was this unimaginable trauma, coupled with other personal stresses and challenges, that were cumulatively more than she could bear. They caused her to reach a point where life was too hard for her to live. Despite her continued courage and long-suffering, Molly's disease, ultimately diagnosed as PTSD, took her life.

We wish Molly could have found the healing she needed to prolong her stay with us here on earth. Our own spiritual faith has helped both Steve and I feel at peace that she is on the other side of the veil, waiting for us until we all will be together again.

After Molly's funeral, many people expressed their gratitude that our family did not "hide" her mental illness and that our openness has genuinely helped them. Perhaps in reading this, you, too, will find the courage not to hide this painful disease. We don't claim to have the answers. After all, Molly's life did not have a good ending, even *with* enduring family support. We do know, however, that many still struggle all around us. Perhaps our willingness to share our story will support and encourage you to speak more openly about mental health.

<u>"LIGHT OVERCOMES DARKNESS"</u> — Allen, Jean's son

After her several days in Hospital 1, I was finally able to reach out to my mom over the phone. It was immediately apparent that her entire reality had shattered—and it was the lowest I had ever heard her. It wasn't long before our conversation spiraled into a truly dark place. She began mumbling things in a lower, deeper voice, telling me how bad she was and how everyone should stay away from her. Not only was it apparent that she was not entirely herself, but it was almost as if she was under the influence of an evil spirit or an overpowering force of thought.

However, it was at that moment that I felt a rush of light come into my mind and heart—a ray of hope made possible through Jesus Christ. I strongly felt that I needed to tell my mom how good she was. I spoke of the many kindnesses she had done for others and reminded her that she was loved by so many. And I assured her of the tremendous support that she had.

I also felt impressed to remind her about the reality of light— and that all light can eventually overcome the darkness. More than anything, I felt strongly to assure her that I believed in the light and power of Jesus Christ. As we spoke, I could literally feel that light consuming the darkness she was experiencing. Confidence surged

85

within me as I internally sensed the inevitable light of my mom's future, a hopeful view of her eventual "good things to come" (Hebrews 9:11).

It was not as though she experienced any remarkable transformation during that call. Still, the tone of her voice reverted to her usual self. I was now speaking with her—the person—and not the darkness. Her throaty, mumbling voice was replaced with a sudden tenor of clarity, as though she'd been "pulled back" from the cavernous despair to which she had descended.

Today it is amazing to see my mom so enveloped in the light first shown to me nearly a decade ago. Bathed in the light of her Savior, she consistently taps into His power. And as promised by Him, there is now an undeniable and living "well of water springing up" inside of her (John 4:14).

I believe that this divine light of hope initiated her release from the darkness.

"NEVER SAY NEVER" — Name Withheld 2

I am writing this anonymously out of respect for our daughter's wish for privacy surrounding her struggles to maintain her mental health. Discovering that our loved ones are suffering from mental illness initially leaves many staggering in unbelief. It did me.

Our daughter was a happy, delightful, well-adjusted child and an exemplary teenager and young adult. She was an excellent athlete, a straight-A, self-motivated student that never gave my husband or me any measure of frustration or anxiety. Her pursuit of excellence earned her a full-ride scholarship to a prestigious university. We felt that any dreams she pursued were solidly within her reach.

During her first year of university, a disturbing mental-health crisis reared its ugly head. Our daughter came home as an altered person during her college break—confused, paranoid, and undeniably debilitated. Her words detailed childhood and young adult memories that had no basis in reality and were truly evil.

For days she stayed awake in a manic state, followed by days of a depression so deep she could barely pull herself out of bed. One night she disappeared. After frantically searching, we found that she had admitted herself into the local hospital for fear she would destroy herself. The awful diagnosis was twofold—bipolar disorder and schizophrenia.

Incredibly, my daughter was able to pull herself together enough during that short holiday week to convince us that she was "good to go" and returned only slightly behind schedule to university to finish out her very demanding studies.

Very soon, however, her world imploded, and so did ours! She disappeared into the back streets of a major U.S. city without a trace. The feelings of guilt my husband and I experienced were totally oppressive. I flew 1600 miles to find her. I went places within that huge and intimidating city that no one should ever risk going. One winter night a week later, I miraculously found her huddled under a park bench. And again, miraculously, I was able to get her on a plane headed for home.

Next followed rounds of stays in various psychiatric hospitals. Though disturbing and stressful for the family, it was more difficult for us when she was not hospitalized. The voices inside her head were still demanding that she act on self-destructive activities that none of us could control. Like many young adults, she was non-compliant when it came to taking her prescription medications preferring street drugs that produced effects more to her liking. Our beautiful daughter was at risk, out of control, and we felt helpless to change anything.

The next twelve years included admittance into more psychiatric hospitals, short periods of stability, followed by longer periods of instability and disappearances. The medical and legal advice was "Stop looking for her," and "Save yourself and the rest of your family."

I was unable and unwilling to follow this advice. I would leave home for weeks at a time, trying to find our daughter in homeless shelters and on the most dangerous back streets, always coaxing her to return home and into treatment programs that, unfortunately, never worked.

My husband held firm to the opinion that my willingness to abandon all else dear to me and to place myself at risk had only negative outcomes. He thought I was merely providing a safety net for our daughter and removing any desire she had to access a significant change of behavior. The discord nearly caused the disintegration of our marriage and family life.

It took me years to realize that you can't help someone to recover who is not invested in that process. I finally told our daughter that if she disappeared again, I would not try to find her.

She did, however, disappear again. I was, of course, heartbroken and anxious beyond belief for her safety. Considering her state of mind, I felt we might never see her again—that she would be just another nameless, faceless person on the streets.

But after more than one year of not knowing where she was, our daughter came home. She was malnourished, unhealthy, and drug-addicted. Mentally, however, she was clear enough to recognize that her self-destructive path would lead to her premature death, and she now had the desire to turn it all around.

We were lucky to obtain a very skilled psychiatrist who could walk her through the initial phase of regaining enough confidence to start rebuilding her life. The mental effort and personal tenacity she displayed were inspiring to watch. The ability of the human spirit to rebound was a complete revelation to me.

I can't tell you how much respect I have for our daughter. I have no idea how she obtained the strength and discipline to do the work, but I am so grateful she did! She has been sober for six years, is self-sufficient, and working to obtain a joyful life. She is very watchful and proactive about protecting and maintaining it. She found a caring therapist whom she trusts with her deepest emotions and fears. We now have a beautiful, rewarding, and mutually supportive relationship that I value beyond words.

I would never consider myself an expert on mental illness, but these are some of the things I personally needed to work on to be of any value in her recovery.

- *First, I had to allow my cherished daughter to resolve her own predicament.* It turns out that making life too easy for her merely reinforced her idea that she had no control over her own life. I now recognize that our daughter chose a better, life-altering trajectory only when I backed away.

- *I had to readjust my expectations.* I had to accept that the lofty dreams my daughter once held for herself were no longer reachable. How devastating for her, and yet how incredible she can still thrive despite that reality.

- *I had to really listen to what my daughter was saying without shock and without judgment.* Her shrunken mental health had left her abandoned on an island with no ability to return to the mainland. She felt terrified, horrified, totally disappointed, and without hope of ever feeling different. I think that her lifeline was knowing that people loved her without condition or even expectation when she could not feel the same way about herself.

- *I had to forgive my daughter for overturning our world as we knew it.* She did not choose to cause the chaos, anger, and anxiety that occurred within our family. Rather, mental illness spun her out of control—and we, too, were pulled into the hurricane along with her. I learned that often those that disappear are misled by the voices in their head that convince them that their friends and family are better off without them.

- *I had to take a hard look at myself and make some personal changes.* Together with my daughter, we went through almost one year of therapeutic counseling. During therapy, I heard things about myself that were difficult to hear and accept. I discovered, often unintentionally, that I was part of the problem. I feel that I came out the other side of this experience as an improved human being with much more empathy and an increased capacity to actually help.

While writing this, I recognize the monumental effort it takes to heal from mental illness, knowing that some of you have lost loved ones along this torturous road. I have the greatest empathy for you. I often pictured that I, too, would one day be dealing with that same emotional aftermath. Or, because of our beautiful daughter's frequent disappearances, we might never know what happened to her if she never returned.

There may be others of you who are grinding through, day-by-day trying to help a loved one with a debilitating mental illness. At this time, you may see no light at the end of the tunnel. I understand that no emotion is left untouched and that you often have no clue what your next move should be. I also clearly recognize the desire to walk away from it all. I challenge you, however, to never give up hope. I can testify that things can change. There are inexplicable, unexpected successes that are ever so sweet.

My advice is this—*Never say never!*

"BALANCING EMPATHY WITH SELF-PROTECTION"
Jared—Jean's son-in-law

Part of me wonders if I should be offering any advice at all since I feel neither qualified to counsel others nor particularly successful at navigating these waters myself. But what I lack in expertise, perhaps I can make up for in experience. At times, I have felt very alone, surrounded by family members in mental health crises, doing my best to stay mentally healthy myself so that I can support those around me. Perhaps that is my most pressing personal takeaway—to do your best to protect and preserve your own mental health—not by closing out others but by staying open to their needs.

As I see family members on their debilitating mental and emotional roller coasters, I have tried to reassure them that I am there on the platform, keeping an eye on them through every loop and drop. I reassure them that I cannot be on the roller coaster with them, or I will never be able to help them when the car comes back to the platform. Balancing self-care with empathy for others and selflessness with self-protection is one of the hardest things to discover (discern), and it requires a lot of self-correction as we try to find a middle ground.

Speaking of balance, I've seen the need to provide as much balance as possible for my loved ones when they are suffering. Balance between what I can do for them and what they must do for themselves. Balance between mercy and justice. Balance between forgiveness and accountability. Balance between gentleness and toughness. People in trauma will need both.

After a particularly devastating bipolar episode, I remember telling my son that every sufferer deserves to have both a pillow and a punching bag but that he must never confuse one for the other. In his case, his mother is the pillow, and I'm the punching bag (thankfully, only metaphorically!), and I reassured him that I was okay playing that role when he needed it. In our case, I'm grateful that my wife and I could combine our gifts to help provide our children with that balance. It's more difficult when the same person has to serve both roles simultaneously, but it's equally important to develop both sides within ourselves. Striving for that balance is key—for their sake and for our own.

"REMEMBERING HER TIME IN THE MENTAL HOSPITAL"
Tom—Jean's brother

All I remember was a phone call. I'm not sure if mom initiated it or if you called. I think mom was with you and maybe handed the phone over to you. It was like I was talking to a zombie. You seemed to be heavily medicated and spoke very softly and slowly. I could barely hear you. I could tell you were having trouble collecting your thoughts or trying to complete a sentence. I knew it was probably severe depression. I had seen it before in my field of work as a firefighter paramedic. I was saddened by what I was hearing. I noticed the pain in your voice and that you really didn't want to talk. When your voice became shaky, you started to cry and quickly ended the conversation. It must have been a horrible experience.

I'm glad you are doing better.

I know our sister Julie has struggled with depression, too. Stress, no matter what the cause, is a killer. Fortunately, you were able to overcome both the stress and the depression!

"MAE'S STORY" — granddaughter of Jean's friend

My name is Mae. I'm 17 years old. And I found a dead body in the desert.

I was riding with my family into the desert to go shooting during our reunion. The dirt road was bumpy, so we drove slow and steady. There, right next to a parked vehicle, right outside my window, I saw a man. He was only in my view for a few seconds as the car jostled by, but the image stayed with me. He was lying on his stomach, so I didn't see his face, but I knew he was dead. He looked older—maybe in his 70's or 80's. There was a pool of blood that looked black around his head. His shirt was lifted a little in the back so that I could see his skin. It was very pale and wrinkly.

I was the only one in the vehicle who noticed. I texted my mom, who was in the car ahead, wondering if she had seen the man's body. I waited for her response. I didn't want to scare my two sisters, my young cousin, and my grandpa, all in the car with me, by saying anything.

I was still terrified by the memory of the sight. I felt it was most likely a suicide but also wondered if the man had instead been murdered. I didn't know what to think. It's an eerie feeling to see a dead body in the middle of the desert.

Everyone else rolled their windows down to get some air, but I kept mine up as if the glass would offer some sort of protection. I kept looking behind the vehicle because I felt paranoid. I was hyperventilating but also trying to keep my feelings a secret. I didn't want anyone else to become afraid.

The drive felt like it took forever, and I just kept replaying what I had witnessed in my head. "Was it really a person?" "Should I keep it a secret?" "Should I wait to see if someone else sees it on our way out?" "Could it have been a mannequin?" "There's no way. He was right there—right by his vehicle, lying in a pool of his blood!" I couldn't deny what my eyes knew to be true.

About fifteen minutes later, we got to our destination in the middle of the desert. I got out of the car and didn't say anything. That's when my mom checked her messages and asked, "Did I see what?" She looked at me with concern. Staring back, I said, "I saw a dead person."

She brought me away from the kids toward the group of adults. She whispered to my dad, "Mae thinks she saw a dead body." My dad then questioned, too loudly, "Mae thinks she saw a dead body?!" My mom shushed him, but I found out later that my sisters overheard.

At this point, I started crying, so I don't remember super clearly what came next, but I'll try my best to describe it. The five grownups talked quickly and quietly about what to do while I received hugs from my mom and aunt. I told them where I had seen the man. My dad and grandpa got in one of the cars to go back and confirm what I saw and contact the authorities. I think they were hoping it was a mannequin or something other than a dead body.

As my mom explained what dad was going to do, I told her, "I know that it was a dead man close to his vehicle. I know it!"

My mom and I walked away from everyone while my aunt supervised the kids. Mom hugged me as she said a prayer for me, for the man, and for the man's family. We prayed for my dad and grandpa, who were on their way to the body. We prayed for the authorities that would be arriving soon to take care of things and those that would be contacting that man's family. It helped me feel peace, but I was still shaken by what I had seen.

About a minute after we finished our prayer, dad texted and said that he and my grandpa were calling 911 and they would be a bit longer. My uncle said that since that road was the only way in and out, he wanted to keep the younger kids oblivious about what was happening. He thought we should go ahead with our desert activity plans. The kids had already seen me crying, but thankfully, there was no way they could guess what had happened.

Soon dad drove back to our site while my grandpa stayed to wait for the authorities. We started shooting for a bit, and I did stop crying even though I kept thinking about what had happened. An hour later, grandpa was back. He walked with me a bit, saying how sorry he was that I had to see that. Dad came over, too, and said the same thing. Of course, I started crying again, but I was worried for my dad and grandpa this time. I didn't see the man's face, and he was only in my line of sight for a few seconds. But my dad and grandpa were specifically looking for a dead body. They had to stay and wait for the police to come. I wondered how traumatized they were.

The rest of the morning was "normal," although it felt weird to act as if nothing had happened. However, the scene never left my mind. Sometimes I would start thinking about it while the whole family was hanging out and just zone out. My sister Kristine (16) said she could tell what I was thinking about.

Later, as we drove home, all signs of the event had been cleaned up. I made a point to sit in the middle seat and not look too closely.

That evening I took a shower. I already sensed my emotions would come out, and, sure enough, that's what happened. I cried harder than I had in a long while. The image of the body kept replaying in my head. I kept thinking about how my dad and grandpa felt. About what drove the victim to suicide. About what his family was feeling. I cried hardest when I thought about why it had to be me. I'm glad it wasn't my little cousin or my younger siblings, but why couldn't it have been an adult? Out of everyone in both cars, why was I the only one who saw what I saw? I was really struggling at that time, and I was mad at God.

Most of my time in the shower was spent sitting on the floor with water running down my body. I focused on what it felt like on my skin rather than dwelling on the events of the day. I tried to keep my crying quiet and waited for my face to look less red. By the time I left the bathroom, you couldn't tell much that I had been crying.

For a time, my mind thought about what I saw that day every second. The first few nights were the hardest when I cried myself to sleep. Today I still think about it, but I'm more at peace.

My mom told me that she thought I had a spiritual experience. I'll admit that I was initially confused and thought the opposite, but after she explained, I began to agree with her. She said we didn't know what that man was going through, but he was clearly hurting. She said he probably did it close to the road because he wanted to be found. When my dad and grandpa went back, they heard a cell phone ringing in his truck. Someone was looking for him. Because I had seen him, his spirit could have peace. His family could have peace. His friends could have peace.

My sister Kristine has been struggling with depression and suicide ideation for a couple of years now. She said she wished more people would talk about their experience coming upon victims of suicide in order to raise awareness of this crisis. After seeing my reaction to finding this deceased man, she said, "I sometimes wondered what it might be like for my family if they found me that way. I figured it might be hard, but that you guys would be okay. But seeing Mae—seeing how hard it's been on her to see someone in that condition whom she didn't know—well, people should talk about that more."

I still don't know why I was the one to find that man's body out of everyone in our group. But I can now truthfully say that I am grateful for this experience. Maybe it happened to me so I could learn a lesson from it. Maybe it happened for me to spread awareness about suicide in an effort to deter others from making that same choice. Maybe it happened to me so that I could relate to other people in my age group who are going through tough situations. Maybe it was to help provide perspective for my sister to encourage her to stay. I don't know. I'm still figuring out all of the possible reasons.

But I do want whoever hears this story and is struggling with suicidal thoughts or depression, or is just having a hard time in life, to know that it will affect people if you leave this earth. There are people who love you and want you here. I know it feels like there aren't those people sometimes, but I promise you there are—even if it's a stranger like I was to that man. I encourage you to reach out to someone you trust and talk to them about it. It will be so worth it for everyone involved.

I love you, and I think about and pray for those who are going through similar situations. I know I had this experience for a reason, even though I don't understand what it is. I know God loves us, even if we get mad at him for the trials he puts us through. I know that life is hard, but I also know we can get through it.

"A SECOND WITNESS" — Mandy, Jean's daughter

I recently ran into a friend at the grocery store who said she had been reading my mom's memoir. Like me, she found reading about my mom's experience touching and inspiring. Her comment was, "I can't believe what Jean had to go through, how sick she got, and you were there to witness it all!" True, I was there to witness it all—both her severe illness and now her radiant wellness. Though I have enough material to write an entire book, I will attempt to share the biggest lessons from her miraculous healing. My experience is meant to be a second witness to what Jean said. It is all true.

My witness of severe mental illness in a beloved family member. The following recollections are of the phone conversations I had with my mom during the time she was in the California hospitals, and I lived in Utah.

My mom left our church seven years earlier, though she had been on a spiritual journey of seeking truth since then. Every once in a while, I would try to share my beliefs with her, encouraging her to return to our faith. Those conversations never went well. So, I didn't know how to respond when my mom told me from the hospital that she had sold her soul to the devil and went to the "dark side." I didn't want to take advantage of her vulnerable state to *push* my religion on her.

During my youth, both she and my dad taught me religious truths about how to respond when you feel Satan's influence. Now, I reasoned that mom already knew the answers. However, she was so disconnected from reality that I didn't know how to engage with her intellectually. As our conversation continued, her desperate situation and despair became apparent, so my self-restraint gave way. I heard myself saying, "Mom, Satan is not as powerful as Jesus Christ. You can cast Satan out. Remember that experience from my mission! Cast him out! It doesn't matter if you already made a deal with the devil. It isn't too late." Her garbled voice, her dark thoughts, and self-loathing made me wonder if my mom was possessed. At that very moment, she surprised me by taking my suggestion and blurted some awkward form of casting Satan out. The concept that deliverance from evil was possible was a buoy to her—a lifesaving device I threw out in a tumultuous sea. She clung to it. But it took several reminders from myself and other siblings when she would go back to that dark place.

During one phone call, she spoke of her hatred of my dad in a voice that was not characteristic of her—it was deep, vehement, and malicious. Instead of taking her words seriously, I responded lightly, this time by joking with her and saying, "That is okay. We have all hated dad at one time or another." (My dad's a phenomenal person but being mad at dad is just part of family life.) My response startled her, even shook her out of it a little, and we both chuckled. That dark voice was now gone, and we continued to talk normally.

In another exchange, again in her altered, menacing voice, now filled with self-loathing, she said she had been a horrible mother. To be honest, I held hurts from being a child in a large family with six other siblings and, later, three half-brothers. My own mother died when I was six years old, and adjusting to Jean, a living human being who became my stepmother, came a year later. Jean did all the work—all the jobs a busy mother often would do. However, our emotional relationship was sometimes hard for me, and I struggled to feel loved.

In my twenties, I often harbored offense and hurt feelings toward Jean. I realized I needed to forgive her even though she had committed no large wrongdoing. I began to pray and ask God to help me forgive her. In time and with maturity, I began to see the situation differently—how impossible her task was, how hard she tried, and how much she gave. No person could ever fill the shoes of my deceased mother nor do what Jean was asked to do perfectly.

No one could ever be enough. It was God who helped me see these things and helped me to forgive.

I was grateful to have done that work years earlier because I responded to my mom sincerely and immediately when she needed me in my thirties. "Now, you listen to me, Mom," I said. "You gave everything that you had to our family. We will never criticize you for not giving more because you gave all that you had. What else could we ask for? What else could be expected?" Mom had no adverse reaction and responded with, "I guess you're right." The conversation was sweet, and I felt the Spirit of God. She thanked me for talking. When I called the following day, she again thanked me, telling me how much that change in narrative helped her. I was so grateful that I had done the work of forgiveness years earlier so that I was able to throw her a lifeline. This experience was one of the many that she doesn't remember from the hospital. I wish she did because, at the time, it was holy for both of us. Personally, I am grateful for it.

You can heal from mental and emotional illness. All the sordid details my mom shares in her book are true. It was so disturbing to see her lose touch with reality and speak in a Satanic-type voice. I didn't know if she would ever get better. I hoped she would be stable but assumed she would always be somewhat depressed or anxious. However, just as real as how sick she got was how well she became. Her recovery happened step by step until she was healthier than I'd ever known her to be. I never expected such miraculous and thorough healing.

Several members of my large family have had moments of struggle with less-than-optimal mental health though none ever got as sick as my mom. However, I have observed mom's excellent mental state and emotional disposition for several years now. I have often thought, "There is no one in our family with better emotional and mental health right now than my mom." Because she "slogged" that difficult road, she has been able to help many of us navigate out of our own dark times. She has gone from being the sickest patient to become the angel who ministers to our family. My mom is serene, gentle, non-judgmental, and compassionate. Her healing has been a miracle and an honor to witness. YOU CAN GET BETTER TOO!

Mental illness is a condition, not the definition of who you are. My mom wasn't crazy—her brain just got sick. This illness of the brain is not often recognized in our society. Spiritual leader Jeffrey R. Holland said this as it relates to mental illness. "However bewildering this all may be, these afflictions are some of the realities of mortal life, and there should be no more shame in acknowledging them than in acknowledging a battle with high blood pressure or the sudden appearance of a malignant tumor."[1]

It is unfair to define people by the symptoms they are experiencing. My mom wasn't her mental illness, and the symptoms she displayed weren't her personality or her eternal nature—they were something she was experiencing.

Mental hospitals are necessary but shouldn't be viewed as the place where you get well mentally. Mental hospitals are similar to emergency rooms in regular hospitals. ERs don't treat cancer, and they are lousy at helping with most medical conditions. However, they are excellent at providing care for accidents, strokes, heart attacks, and trauma. You go there to get stabilized, not usually healed.

In general, my family doesn't love mental hospitals after seeing what my mom and others in our family have gone through. However, they serve a definite purpose. Psychiatric hospitals help stabilize a person on medications and provide a safe environment when a person is at risk of harming themselves. For that, we are grateful. But my mom's healing didn't happen at that stage, and no amount of talk therapy was helpful when she was psychotic.

HER PATH TO HEALING

My mom healed in all the areas that produce a whole person—biopsychosocial/spiritual.

Biological Healing - My mom needed powerful psychiatric medications to help stabilize her, and she needed assistance to sleep. Sleep is vital to overcoming mental illness. As she described, the psychiatric and medication road was not smooth, but it was essential to stabilize her. Some years later, mom no longer needed the medicine or therapy that her psychiatrist and therapist once administered.

Juicing and consuming a more plant-based diet were very powerful things she did to heal her physical body. She came alive. I saw it. We all did. And so, we all chugged down those vile fresh-pressed vegetable juice combinations with her because we wanted to feel that same vitality. I learned to love those juices—especially celery!

Psychological Healing - This stage typically happens in therapy. However, not all the treatment my mom had earlier in her life was helpful or healing. Before her hospitalizations, I had reservations about the therapist my mom had seen for several years, and I felt that the therapy she then obtained was harming her. However, the treatment my mom received from the new therapist *after* the mental hospital was very beneficial. That clinician helped my mom feel loved, validated, and accepted. Her form of "relational therapy" grounded my mom. And though better, I did observe that mom was still depressed, and her psychological work would continue after this therapist moved out of the area.

Mom's second clinician had a slightly different therapeutic approach. She gently pushed mom to try different "doing" things during the week, challenging her to make changes. Mom didn't embrace all of this therapist's modalities, but this change in method, in my opinion, had a tremendous impact.

One important offering was meditation. I saw the practice of Mindfulness Meditation transform my mom and bring her to a state of more wholeness and wellness than I had ever witnessed before in her.

Social Healing - My mom initially isolated herself from people and places. Part of her becoming well meant not doing that anymore. She started by reconnecting with my dad, her mom, our family, and eventually, old friends. She rebuilt hurt relationships. Her church community contributed to her social healing. I saw her confidence grow as she excelled in the workplace and watched her hone new skills during employment. It did not happen overnight—

this all took time. Presently, service to others has become the hallmark of her wellness.

Spiritual Healing - I believe that the most powerful healing came when my mom turned to God and reconciled with Him. However, her becoming well was not as simplistic as having faith and praying. Those were steps in the right direction; God guided her to heal in the many mentioned areas. I believe God was the source of all the good things that happened.

Be compassionate with yourself and others who are struggling. In this book, my mom shared very little of her backstory. If she had, I think the most common response would be, "Of course she went crazy! It is a marvel that it didn't happen sooner." When first married, Jean was very high functioning, living a demanding life that few others could. She was stepmom to seven, mother to three more, and wife to a very busy business owner and church leader. Over time, however, her reserves wore down. During her late 40s into her 50s, she started dealing with her childhood, including her own parent-child relationships. I found her focus interesting because she was so much farther away from her childhood at that point. She thought about her dad a lot. In my opinion, her father's berating voice from her childhood, now a permanent resident in her mind, got louder. I don't know if, at that age, life slowed down enough for her to deal with these issues or if it just caught with her. But I have seen this pattern in other women of that age group. It makes me wonder if this is one of the stages of midlife. Looking at the past may be one of the tasks you work on at that age.

When a loved one is struggling with depression, don't take their irritability, annoyance, anger, and rejection personally. I've witnessed other family members struggle with mental health. Like Jean, their initial presenting symptoms are annoyance and anger. Typically, the receiver of their displeasure interprets this as a rejection of themselves or hatred towards them. It's hard not to take it personally. When someone is struggling, it's usually themselves that they actually hate. Often, they are not aware of it. Try not to take it personally. My advice is to love.

Family relationships can heal. One of the biggest fallouts for families dealing with a mental health crisis is harmed relationships. As stated above, when people are hurting, they tend to hurt others around them. I am grateful to report that relationships in our family that once were incredibly hard have now turned into the sweetest associations. Our family has healed, and so can yours!

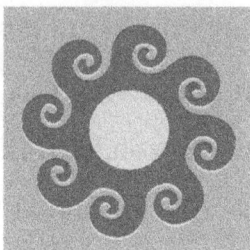

Chapter 11

AMERICAN FOUNDATION FOR SUICIDE PREVENTION (AFSP)

"What leads to suicide?" you ask.

According to the American Foundation for Suicide Prevention (AFSP), there's no single cause for suicide. Suicide most often occurs when stressors and health issues converge to create an experience of hopelessness and despair. Depression is the most common condition associated with suicide, and it is often undiagnosed and untreated. Conditions like depression, anxiety, and substance use problems, especially when unaddressed, increase risk for suicide. Yet it is important to note that most people who actively manage their mental health conditions go on to engage in life.[1]

The Centers for Disease Control and Prevention (CDC) Data & Statistics Fatal Injury Report for 2020 states that suicide is the **12th leading cause of death** in the United States.[2]

45,979 Americans died by suicide in 2020. • It's the **3rd** leading cause of death for ages 10-19 • It's the **2nd** leading cause of death for ages 20-34. It's the **4th** leading cause of death for ages 35-44. **Over one-third** of people who died by suicide were 55 or older.

10% of adult Americans have thoughts about suicide.

1.2 million Americans attempted suicide.

54% of Americans have been affected by suicide in some way.

Men died by suicide **3.9x** more often than females. Females are **1.8x** more likely to attempt suicide.

54% of firearm deaths were suicides. **53%** of all suicides were by firearms.

In 2019, the suicide rate was **1.5x higher for Veterans** than for non-Veteran adults over the age of 18.

90% of those who die by suicide had a diagnosable mental health condition at the time of their death.

46% of Americans ages 18+ living with a mental health condition received treatment in the past year.

72% of communities in the United States did not have enough mental health providers to serve residents in 2021, according to federal guidelines.

RISK FACTORS are characteristics or conditions that increase the chance that a person may take their life.₃ They include:

Health

Mental health conditions:

- Depression
- Substance use problems
- Bipolar disorder
- Schizophrenia
- Personality traits of aggression, mood changes, and poor relationships
- Conduct disorder

Anxiety disorders (PTSD)

Serious physical health conditions, including pain

Traumatic brain injury

Environmental

- Access to lethal means, including firearms and drugs
- Prolonged stress such as harassment, bullying, relationship problems, or unemployment
- Stressful life events, like rejection, divorce, financial crisis, other life transitions, or loss
- Exposure to another person's suicide or to graphic or sensationalized accounts of suicide

Historical

- Previous suicide attempts
- Family history of suicide
- Childhood abuse, neglect, or trauma

Protective Factors

- Access to mental healthcare and being proactive about mental health
- Feeling connected to family and community support
- Problem-solving and coping skills
- Limited access to lethal means
- Cultural and religious beliefs that encourage connecting and help-seeking, discourage suicidal behavior, or create a strong sense of purpose or self-esteem

Warning Signs

Something to look out for when concerned that a person may be suicidal is a change in behavior or the presence of entirely new behaviors. This is of sharpest concern if the new or changed behavior is related to a painful event, loss, or change. Most people who take their lives exhibit one or more warning signs, either through what they say or what they do.

Talk

If a person talks about:

- Killing themselves
- Feeling hopeless
- Having no reason to live
- Being a burden to others
- Feeling trapped
- Unbearable pain

Behavior

Behaviors that may signal risk, especially if related to a painful event, loss, or change:

- Increased use of alcohol or drugs
- Looking for a way to end their lives, such as searching online for methods
- Withdrawing from activities
- Isolating from family and friends
- Sleeping too little or too much
- Visiting or calling people to say goodbye
- Giving away prized possessions
- Aggression
- Fatigue

Mood

People who are considering suicide often display one or more of the following moods:

- Depression
- Anxiety
- Loss of interest
- Irritability
- Humiliation/Shame

- Agitation/Anger
- Relief/Sudden Improvement

What to do when someone is at risk[4]

If you think someone is thinking about suicide, assume you are the only one who will reach out. Here's how to talk to someone who may be struggling with their mental health.

Have an honest conversation

1. Talk to them in private
2. Listen to their story
3. Tell them you care about them
4. Ask directly if they are thinking about suicide
5. Encourage them to seek treatment or contact their doctor or therapist
6. Avoid debating the value of life, minimizing their problems, or giving advice

IF YOU'RE CONCERNED ABOUT SOMEONE

Talk in Private

Listen to their story and let them know you care. Ask directly about suicide calmly and without judgment. Show understanding and take their concerns seriously. Let them know their life matters to you. That one conversation could save a life.

121

If A Person Says They Are Thinking About Suicide, Take The Person Seriously.

Someone considering suicide is experiencing a life-threatening health crisis and may not believe they can be helped. Work with them to keep them safely away from lethal means like firearms and drugs and remind them that their suffering is temporary.

Stay with them and call the National Suicide Prevention Lifeline:

<u>1-800-273-TALK (8255)</u>

Be sure to follow up with them after the crisis to see how they're doing.

IF YOU'RE STRUGGLING

Don't Wait for Someone to Reach Out
Seek mental health treatment or tell your clinician about your suicidal thinking.

Treat yourself like you would treat someone else who needs your help.

HEALING CONVERSATIONS

Personal Support for Suicide Loss[5]

Healing Conversations gives those who have lost someone to suicide the opportunity to talk with experienced AFSP volunteers. These volunteers, who are themselves survivors of suicide loss, offer understanding and guidance in the weeks and months following a suicide death.

Available in person, on the phone, or by video chat, AFSP volunteers are familiar with the isolation that so often accompanies a death of this kind and are able to show suicide loss survivors a way forward into a world of support, by creating an opportunity for the newly bereaved to speak openly with, and ask questions of, someone who has been there, too, and truly gets it.

You can fill out an AFSP Healing Conversations request form to speak with someone.[6]

MISSION[7]

The American Foundation for Suicide Prevention (AFSP) is dedicated to saving lives and bringing hope to those affected by suicide.

AFSP creates a culture that's smart about mental health by engaging in the following core strategies:

- Funding scientific research
- Educating the public about mental health and suicide prevention
- Advocating for public policies in mental health and suicide prevention
- Supporting survivors of suicide loss and those affected by suicide

American Foundation for Suicide Prevention website: https://afsp.org/

Chapter 12

THERE IS HOPE!

"The people that walked in darkness have seen a great light: they that dwell in the land of the shadow of death, upon them hath the light shined." *(Isaiah 9:2)*

"Every day do something to help someone even if it is something small. As you figure out how to help others, it will force you to start thinking in a positive way." (Dandapani, Weekend Reflection email, 9/12/20)

"Blessed are ye that weep now: for ye shall laugh." *(Luke 6:21)*

"It doesn't help someone battered by a storm to hear that summer's coming. It does help, though, if a friend will help hold the umbrella or keep us company as the wind howls. " (Lois M. Collins, *Deseret News National Edition*, April 19, 2015)

"Know ye not that ye are in the hands of God?" *(Mormon 5:23)*

"Illness of any kind, as evidenced by any physical or emotional problems, is simply blocked or stuck energy, *chi* that has gotten withheld from the general flow, tipping the body-mind out of balance." (Belleruth Naparstek, *Staying Well with Guided Imagery: How to Harness the Power of Your Imagination for Health and Healing*, 54)

"Learn of me, and listen to my words; walk in the meekness of my Spirit, and you shall have peace in me." (D&C 19:23)

"That which we persist in doing becomes easier to do, not that the nature of the thing has changed, but our power to do so is increased." (Ralph Waldo Emerson)

"This I know; for God is for me." (Psalm 56:9)

"The patience that develops with meditation ceases after a while to be patience at all." (David Fontana, *The Elements of Meditation*, 50)

"For God hath not given us the spirit of fear; but of power, and of love, and of a sound mind." (2 Timothy 1:7)

"No pain that we suffer, no trial that we experience is wasted. It ministers to our education, to the development of such qualities of patience, faith, fortitude, and humility…It is through sorrow and suffering, toil and tribulation, that we gain the education that we come (to earth) to acquire and which will make us more like our Father and Mother in heaven." (Elder Orson F. Whitney, *We Believe: Doctrines and Principles of the Church of Jesus Christ of Latter-Day Saints*, book by Rulon T. Burton, 10)

"By small and simple things are great things brought to pass; and small means in many instances doth confound the wise." *(Alma 37:6)*

"The best way to find out what we really need is to get rid of what we don't." (Marie Kondo, *www.konmari.com*)

"Look unto me in every thought; doubt not, fear not." *(D&C 6:36)*

"Life isn't about avoiding the bruises. It's about collecting the scars to prove we showed up for it." (Iman Bowie, tweeting right before her husband, David Bowie, passed away. *https://twitter.com/The_Real_IMAN/status/685448175281418240*)

"Be strong and of a good courage, fear not, nor be afraid of them: for the LORD thy God, he it is that doth go with thee; he will not fail thee nor forsake thee." *(Deuteronomy 31:6)*

"As soon as you become aware that your thoughts are having a negative effect, ask yourself, 'Would I deliberately choose these thoughts?' If the answer is no, you can substitute a positive affirmation every time negative thoughts arise." (Goldstein and Soares, *The Joy Within*, 34)

"For now we see through a glass darkly; but then face to face: now I know in part; but then shall I know even as also I am known." (1 Corinthians 13:12)

"God takes the long-view, and our ultimate good may mean short-term pain, confusion, or heartache." (Jeffrey S. McClellan, *Thy Troubles to Bless*, BYU Lecture Series, June 10, 2018)

"But behold, he did deliver them because they did humble themselves before him; and because they cried mightily unto him he did deliver them out of bondage; and thus doth the Lord work with his power in all cases among the children of men, extending the arm of mercy towards them that put their trust in him." (Mosiah 29:20)

"Face the fear and do it anyway." (Joshua Rosenthal, *Increase Your Confidence*, Institute for Integrative Nutrition Health Coach Program, Module 39, 2017)

"And now, verily I say unto you, and what I say unto one I say unto all, be of good cheer, little children; for I am in your midst, and I have not forsaken you." (D&C 61:36)

"Since all potentials in the fifth dimension known as the quantum (or the unified field) exist in the eternal present moment, the only way you can create a new life, heal your body, or change your predictable future is to get beyond yourself." (Dr. Joe Dispenza, *Becoming Supernatural*, xxiv-xxv)

"I waited patiently for the LORD; and he inclined unto me, and heard my cry. He brought me up also out of an horrible pit, out of the miry clay, and set my feet upon a rock, and established my goings. And he hath put a new song in my mouth, even praise unto our God: many shall see it, and fear, and shall trust in the LORD." (Psalm 40:1-3)

"Darkness cannot drive out darkness: only light can do that." (Martin Luther King, Jr. and James M. Washington, *A Testament of Hope: The Essential Writings and Speeches by Martin Luther King Jr.)*

"And he said to the woman, Thy faith hath saved thee; go in peace." (Luke 7:50)

"Emotion, which is suffering, ceases to be suffering as soon as we form a clear and precise picture of it." (Baruch Spinoza, *Man's Search for Meaning*, book by Victor E. Frankl, 98)

"The Lord did hear their cries, and did strengthen them." *(Alma 2:28)*

"Sharing stories about depression is the best, first step in fighting both the disease itself and the stigma that surrounds it." (Jane Clayson Johnson, *Silent Souls Weeping—Depression: Sharing Stories of Hope, 196*)

"Remember the worth of souls is great in the sight of God." *(D&C 18:10)*

"True justice is paying only once for each mistake. True injustice is paying more than once for each mistake." (Don Miguel Ruiz, *The Four Agreements: A Toltec Wisdom Book*, 14)

"Trust in the Lord with all thine heart; and lean not unto thine own understanding. In all thy ways acknowledge him, and he shall direct thy paths." *(Proverbs 3:5-6)*

"Focus not on what I can't do but rather on what I can do." (Gary E. Stevenson, "Plain and Precious Truths," *Ensign Magazine*, November 2015)

"Come ye yourself apart into a desert place, and rest a while." (Mark 6:31)

"Sometimes we can simply observe the inner turmoil and abide it, rather than hardening to it." (Jacob Z. Hess, et.al, *The Power of Stillness: Mindful Living for Latter-Day Saints*, 69)

"And I will also ease the burdens which are put upon your shoulders, that even you cannot feel them upon your backs, even while you are in bondage; and this will I do that ye may stand as witnesses for me hereafter, and that ye may know of a surety that I, the Lord God, do visit my people in their afflictions." (Mosiah 24:14)

"We need to embrace our fear, hatred, anguish, and anger.... We stop running from our pain. With all our courage and tenderness, we recognize, acknowledge, and identify it." (Thich Nhat Hanh, *The Heart of the Buddha's Teaching: Transforming Suffering into Peace, Joy, and Liberation*, 29)

"Be patient in afflictions, for thou shalt have many; but endure them, for lo, I am with thee, even unto the end of thy days." (D&C 24:8)

"God, give us grace to accept with serenity the things that cannot be changed, courage to change the things that should be

changed, and the wisdom to distinguish the one from the other."
(Elisabeth Sifton, *The Serenity Prayer: Faith and Politics in Times of Peace and War*, 6)

"So I will be with thee: I will not fail thee, nor forsake thee." (Joshua 1:5)

"Our deepest fear is not that we are inadequate. Our deepest fear is that we are powerful beyond measure. It is our light, not our darkness that most frightens us…. As we are liberated from our own fear, our presence automatically liberates others." (Marianne Williamson, *A Return to Love: Reflections on the Principles of A COURSE IN MIRACLES*, 190-191)

"For the Lamb which is in the midst of the throne shall feed them, and shall lead them unto living fountains of waters: and God shall wipe away all tears from their eyes." (Revelation 7:17)

"There is nothing more important to true growth than realizing that you are not the voice of the mind—you are the one who hears it." (Michael Singer, *The Untethered Soul,* 12)

"Thou knowest the greatness of God; and he shall consecrate thine afflictions for thy gain." (2 Nephi 2:2)

"Come what may, and love it." (Elder Joseph B. Wirthlin, *Ensign Magazine*, November 2008, 26)

"Wherefore, I now send upon you another Comforter, even upon you my friends, that it may abide in your hearts, even the Holy Spirit of promise." (D&C 88:3)

"If we can uproot our constant, frantic tendency to want things to be different, then we can bring an end to the pain and suffering that that tendency constantly creates." (Will Johnson, *The Posture of Meditation: A Practical Manual for Meditators of All Traditions*, 14)

"For I have satiated the weary soul, and I have replenished every sorrowful soul." (Jeremiah 31:25)

"You are not your mind." (Eckhart Tolle, *The Power of Now: A Guide to Spiritual Enlightenment*, 11)

"And he said unto me, My grace is sufficient for thee; for my strength is made perfect in weakness. Most gladly therefore will I rather glory in my infirmities that the power of Christ may rest upon me. Therefore I take pleasure in infirmities, in reproaches, in necessities, in persecutions, in distress for Christ's sake: for when I am weak, then I am strong." (2 Corinthians 12:9-10)

"Practice makes permanent." (Goldie Hawn and Wendy Holden, *10 Mindful Minutes: Giving Our Children—and Ourselves—the Social and Emotional Skills to Reduce Stress and Anxiety for Healthier, Happier Lives*, 68)

"For, behold, I have refined thee, I have chosen thee in the furnace of affliction." (1 Nephi 20:10)

"A thought is harmless unless we believe it. It's not our thoughts, but the attachment to our thoughts, that causes suffering." (Byron Katie, *Loving What Is: Four Questions That Can Change Your Life*, 5)

"I am calm as a summer's morning." (D&C 135:4)

"Many of our emotional and spiritual problems begin, not so much because of difficult experiences, or traumatic experiences of the past, or because there's something inherently wrong with us, but rather because of the way we have learned to use our mind." (M. Catherine Thomas, *The God SEED: Probing the Mystery of Spiritual Development*, 198)

"The LORD lift up his countenance upon thee, and give thee peace." (Numbers 6:26)

"It is a big step toward reclaiming our lives when we realize that, no matter what their content, good, bad, or ugly, we do not have to take our thoughts personally." (Jon Kabat-Zinn, *Mindfulness for Beginners: reclaiming the present moment—and your life*, 39)

"I will not leave you comfortless: I will come to you." (John 14:8)

"Human life is beset with sorrow until we know how to tune in with the Divine Will, whose 'right course' is often baffling to the egoistic intelligence." (Swami Sri Yuktesar, *Autobiography of a Yogi*, book by Paramahansa Yogananda, 168)

"But behold, the Lord hath redeemed my soul from hell; I have beheld his glory, and I am encircled about eternally in the arms of his love." (2 Nephi 1:15)

"We join spokes together in a wheel, but it is the center hole that makes the wagon move. We shape clay into a pot, but it is the emptiness inside that holds whatever we want. We hammer wood for a house, but it is the inner space that makes it livable. We work with being, but non-being is what we use." (Lao-tzu, *Tao Te Ching: A New English Version*, Translation by Stephen Mitchell, 11)

"Peace be unto thy soul; thine adversity and thine afflictions shall be but a small moment." (D&C 121:7)

"You are not your emotions, you are not your limiting beliefs, and you are not darkness. The true you is light and truth." (Brooke Snow, *Living in Your True Identity: Discover, Embrace, and Develop Your Own Divine Nature*, 27)

"Peace be both to thee, and peace be to thine house, and peace be unto all that thou hast." (1 Samuel 25:6)

"There is no such thing as a stressful situation, only stressful responses to a given situation." (The Vedas, *Stress Less, Accomplish More: Meditation for Extraordinary Performance*, book by Emily Fletcher, 45)

"Glory to God in the highest, and on earth peace, good will to men." (Luke 2:14)

"It is only when you have been broken down mentally, emotionally, or spiritually and choose to stand up and keep moving that you can know the true meaning and value of trust." (Iyanla Vanzant, *Trust: Mastering The Four Essential Trusts*, xii)

"And may the Lord bless your soul, and receive you at the last day in his kingdom, to sit down in peace." (Alma 38:15)

"In reality, we are divinity in disguise, and the gods and goddesses in embryo that are contained within us seek to be fully materialized." (Deepak Chopra, *The Seven Spiritual Laws of Success: A Practical Guide to the Fulfillment of Your Dreams*, 3)

"For if they never should have bitter they could not know the sweet." (D&C 29:39)

"I love and approve of myself. I live in the totality of possibility. There is always another way. I am safe. I now go beyond any fears and limitations. I create a new life with new rules that totally support me. I am willing to change." (Jean Stoddard's affirmation, using new thought patterns that negate *anxiety, depression, and suicide,* compiled from the book, *You Can Heal Your Life* by Louise Hay)

TAKEAWAYS

There are many roads to wellness. Therapy, pharmacology, positive affirmations, nutrition, and meditation were some of the many vital steps that helped me heal from depression. Your road may look very different, but the trek you are on is worth completing. "Fresh courage take" (from the hymn, *Come, Come Ye Saints*), and may God bless your every step. There truly is hope!

Jean Conley Stoddard

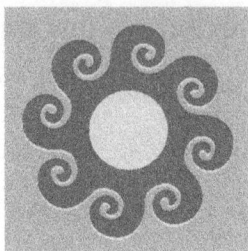

APPENDIX A: CHURCH TALK (APRIL 2015)

Below you will read a talk I gave at Church on April 26, 2015. In my journal, I wrote, *"Gave my first talk since I returned to church—a personal talk focusing on my depression and returning to church, but I think with a hopeful message about belief in Jesus and hope."*

*Good morning, Brothers and Sisters. I'm Sister Jean Stoddard. My husband Rick and I have lived in Penryn for over 31 years. In fact, Rick has lived in Penryn a few years longer than that. For those who don't know, 31 years ago, I married a man with seven children, and over time we added three more. NOW, all our children and 24 grandchildren live all over the country, and we **BOTH** find it rather sad that no one lives in California. So, we do a lot of traveling. However, one of our children—Johnny and his wife Stacy, their daughter Avey, and their soon-to-be-born little one— will be living with us for a year. You will all enjoy knowing them in our ward come July.*

On an even more personal note, many of you may not know that I carry a heavy burden by living on a weekly, daily, and hourly basis with clinical depression. It's the kind that Elder Jeffrey R.

Holland spoke of during his October 2013 General Conference talk when he said, "When I speak of this, I am not speaking of bad hair days, tax deadlines, or other discouraging moments we all have. Everyone is going to be anxious or downhearted on occasion. The Book of Mormon says Ammon and his brethren were depressed at a very difficult time, and so can the rest of us be. But today I am speaking of something more serious, of an affliction so severe that it significantly restricts a person's ability to function fully, a crater in the mind so deep that no one can responsibly suggest it would surely go away if those victims would just square their shoulders and think more positively— though I am a vigorous advocate of square shoulders and positive thinking! No, this dark night of the mind and spirit is more than mere discouragement."[1]

Clinical depression—in 2011, I was even hospitalized with it. For me, in many ways, depression has knocked me flat. I am, as the title to Elder Holland's talk suggests, "Like a Broken Vessel."

On another personal note, some of you might not know that I formally left the Church of Jesus Christ of Latter-day Saints many years before—wrote a letter to Church Leaders in Salt Lake City and resigned my membership. I returned in 2012 though not strong, utterly frightened by my experience in the hospital, and humbled to my core. Again, October 2013 General Conference spoke to me in the form of President Dieter F. Uchtdorf, whose talk "Come, Join with Us" touched my heart. He said, "The search for truth has led millions of people to The Church of Jesus Christ of Latter-Day Saints. However, there are some who leave the Church they once loved. One might ask, 'If the gospel is so wonderful, why would anyone leave?' Sometimes we assume it is because they have been offended or lazy or sinful. Actually, it is not that simple. In fact, there is not just one reason that applies to the variety of situations."[2]

There stood President Uchtdorf, who gave no indication that leaving the Church (which, in my case, had much to do with doubts) was some sort of lack on my part. I loved him for it.

Clinical depression, struggles with doubts, faith, or the lack of faith—these are some burdens I bear. My experience living with these burdens looks like this:

*First, I don't really feel the spirit. The stirred feelings that **you** get enabling **you** to come up here and bear testimony or the inspired thoughts that come into **your** mind or heart to act upon or react to something, well, those things are so much harder for me to feel. Depression masks the spirit. That is why Jesus's lament on the cross, "My God, My God, why hast Thou forsaken me?"(Mark 15:34), can feel like my own reality. And the child's prayer-song,*

"Heavenly Father, are you really there?" rings true. So, what do I do? I borrow testimony from my family. I borrow Loomis 3rd ward's testimony. I borrow those of our church leaders, including Jeffrey R. Holland's. He told me, he told us that we could during the April 2013 conference when he said, "What was once a tiny seed of belief for me has grown into the tree of life, so if your faith is a little tested in this or any season, I invite you to lean on mine."3

My second such experience living with these burdens is that reading the scriptures can be painful. Elder Holland speaks of "faithfully pursuing the time-tested devotional practices that bring the Spirit of the Lord into your life." And one such practice that typically comes to mind is reading the scriptures. But for me, with depression, it's hard to hear many scriptural messages because they can be so firm, harsh, or even fearsome. Reading themes such as "judging of your iniquities," or "falling into transgression," or "becoming ripe for destruction" are hard to hear with depression. And I'm not saying that we aren't to take them to mind and heart and learn from them. But somehow, depression magnifies the pain of these themes.

So, what do I do? I have been counseled by a kind former bishop and by two therapists to make a compilation of scriptures that are uplifting and reassuring for me. And it takes a while to find them.

But they do exist, such as Matthew 11:28, "Come unto me, all ye that labor and are heavy laden, and I will give you rest. Or D&C 50:16, "I will be merciful unto you; he that is weak among you hereafter shall be made strong." Or Psalm 55:4, "In God I will praise his word; in God I have put my trust."

My third experience with depression, doubts, or faith is that there is very little I **KNOW** *to be true—with exception—in the mental hospital, there was something I did come to* **know** *for myself that Satan is real. That there truly exists a dark side. That one can invite him in. And that knowledge terrifies me. I'm still suffering from that experience. But, in fact, it is what scared me straight. It brought me back to the only place I could think to go where there existed its opposite—Jesus Christ. And with that, the only Church I had experience in holding him up most prominently as my Savior and Redeemer.*

Brothers and Sisters, I do hope and do believe that Jesus is the Christ, the son of the living God. Elder Holland has said, "belief is a precious word, an even more precious act, and he need never apologize for 'only believing.' Christ himself, in Mark 5:36, said," Be not afraid, only believe." Alma, in Alma 32:27, said, "Even if ye can no more than desire to believe, let this desire work in you even until ye believe." And Nephi in 2 Nephi 33:10 said, "Hearken unto these words and believe in Christ; and if ye believe not in these words, believe in Christ. And if ye shall believe in Christ ye will believe in these words, for they are the words of Christ, and he hath given them unto me; and they teach all men that they should do good."

On a more proactive note, my fourth experience, especially as it relates to depression, is having done as Elder Holland suggests— sought the counsel of those who hold keys for my spiritual well- being, like the bishop. I have asked for cherished priesthood blessings. I take the Sacrament every week and hold fast to the perfecting promises of the Atonement of Jesus Christ. I am reminded by him to not vote against the preciousness of life by ending it though I, myself, have wanted the pain to be over.

On a more remedial level, I do take medication prescribed by a valued psychiatrist and see weekly a trusted therapist who gives me careful and responsible counsel.

Brothers and Sisters (and I am borrowing from my therapist's words)—I have had crushing blows to my psyche. I've been to hell's door and seen Satan. My eyes have been opened in a way I wouldn't wish on anyone. I have been broken, harmed, and have experienced the dark night of the soul. I'm still in it. It is still hard. The questions come, "Why me? How much more can I tolerate?"

But even then, I realize that I am part of both a family and a church family that have taken me back—even accepted me back. Your faith gives me hope. Indeed, I have friends and family who have loved me back, including my dear mother, who nursed me back to health. I am so grateful.

In the Garden of Gethsemane, Jesus "went a little further, and fell on his face, and prayed, saying, O my Father, if it be possible, let this cup pass from me: nevertheless, not as I will, but as thou wilt." (Matthew 26:39). And so, too, there is Jesus! I did not, nor could I take on, the holy burden of the world's sins and infirmities. All I have is a hope, a belief that he did do that. He did that for us. He did that for me. And because he did, he understands when I feel more hopeless than hopeful.

"Surely, He hath borne our griefs, and carried our sorrows; yet we did esteem him stricken, smitten of God, and afflicted...and with His stripes we are healed." (Isaiah 53:4-5).

In the name of Jesus Christ. Amen.

NOTES

FOREWORD
1. Psalm 23:4 Yea, though I walk through the valley of the shadow of death, I will fear no evil: for thou *art* with me; thy rod and thy staff comfort me.

CHAPTER 1: DEPRESSION'S HARSH REALITY
1. NASA, "*What are Hurricanes?*," September 3, 2014, https://www.nasa.gov/audience/forstudents/k-4/stories/nasa-knows/what-are-hurricanes-k4.html
2. Caribbean Tsunami Formation Center, "*What Type of Tsunamis Exist?*", https://www.ctic.ioc-unesco.org/faq-main/131-what-types-of-tsunamis-exist
3. Dr. Gloria Willcox, "*The Feeling Wheel*," May 8, 2007, https://fwschool.s3.amazonaws.com/Feelings-Wheel-Color.pdf

CHAPTER 2: ENTRANCE TO THE VALLEY OF THE SHADOW OF DEATH
1. California Legislative Information, Welfare and Institutions Code, Division 5 Community and Mental Health Services, https://leginfo.legislature.ca.gov/faces/codes_displaySection.xhtml?lawCode=WIC&sectionNum=5150
2. Utah Code Title 62A Chapter 15 Part A Section 629 https://le.utah.gov/xcode/Title62A/Chapter15/62A-15-S629.html#:~:text=Temporary%20commitment%20%2D%2D%20Requirements%20and%20procedures%20%2D%2D%20Rights.,-(1)&text=provides%20a%20statement%20of%20the,or%20mental%20health%20officer's%20attention
3. Dictionary.com https://www.dictionary.com/browse/psychosis
4. Tia Ghose, "*Robin Williams' Death: What is Lewy Body Dementia?*," Live Science, November 3, 2015, https://www.livescience.com/52682-what-is-lewy-body-dementia.html
5. NeuroStar Advanced Therapy for Mental Health, https://neurostar.com/
6. Alpha-Stim, https://www.alpha-stim.com/
7. Brain-Tap, https://braintap.com/#a_aid=2004MXLE

CHAPTER 5: THE IMPORTANCE OF GOOD PHARMACOLOGY
1. Smitha Bhandari, MD, "*Depression Medications (Antidepressants),*" WebMD, April 14, 2020, https://www.webmd.com/depression/guide/depression-medications-antidepressants
2. U.S. Department of Health and Human Services, U.S. Food and Drug Administration, "*Drugs@FDA: FDA-Approved Drugs,*" https://www.accessdata.fda.gov/scripts/cder/daf/index.cfm

CHAPTER 6: THE IMPORTANCE OF EXCEPTIONAL NUTRITION
1. Physicians Committee for Responsible Medicine, "*21-Day Vegan Kickstart,*" https://kickstart.pcrm.org/en
2. Joe Cross, "*Why Juice?*", https://www.rebootwithjoe.com/juicing/
3. Environmental Working Group, "*EWG's 2023 Shopper's Guide to Pesticides in Produce,*" 2023, https://www.ewg.org/foodnews/summary.php
4. Adda Bjarnadottir, MS, RDN (Ice), "*How to Read Food Labels Without Being Tricked,*" August 19, 2020, https://www.healthline.com/nutrition/how-to-read-food-labels#ingredients-list
5. Jeffrey Smith and Amy Hart, "*Secret Ingredients,*" 2018; 24-hour rental: https://education.knowewell.com/#/online-courses/916707d1-d712-496a-9ad6-27229bded631   Lifetime Access: https://education.knowewell.com/#/online-courses/8304a7e6-1b2c-4bb1-a9a8-c9a3971e13a8

CHAPTER 10: REPORTS FROM THE FRONT LINE
1. Jeffrey R. Holland, "*Like a Broken Vessel,*" Ensign, November 2013 https://www.churchofjesuschrist.org/study/ensign/2013/11/saturday-afternoon-session/like-a-broken-vessel?lang=eng

CHAPTER 11: AMERICAN FOUNDATION FOR SUICIDE PREVENTION (AFSP)
1. American Foundation for Suicide Prevention, "*Risk factors, protective factors, and warning signs,*" https://afsp.org/risk-factors-protective-factors-and-warning-signs
2. American Foundation for Suicide Prevention, "*Suicide statistics,*" https://afsp.org/suicide-statistics/
3. American Foundation for Suicide Prevention, "*Risk factors, protective factors, and warning signs,*" https://afsp.org/risk-factors-protective-factors-and-warning-signs

4. American Foundation for Suicide Prevention, *"What to do when someone is at risk,"* https://afsp.org/what-to-do-when-someone-is-at-risk
5. American Foundation for Suicide Prevention, *"Healing Conversations,"* https://afsp.org/healing-conversations#reach-out-to-a-local-coordinator
6. American Foundation for Suicide Prevention, *"Healing Conversations Request Form,"* https://afsp.wufoo.com/forms/healing-conversations-request-form/
7. American Foundation for Suicide Prevention, *"Mission,"* https://afsp.org/about-afsp#mission

APPENDIX A: CHURCH TALK (APRIL 2015)

1. Jeffrey R. Holland, *"Like a Broken Vessel,"* Ensign, November 2013, https://www.churchofjesuschrist.org/study/ensign/2013/11/saturday-afternoon-session/like-a-broken-vessel?lang=eng
2. Dieter F. Uchtdorf, *"Come, Join with Us,"* Ensign, November 2013, https://www.churchofjesuschrist.org/study/ensign/2013/11/saturday-morning-session/come-join-with-us?lang=eng
3. Jeffrey R. Holland, *"Lord, I Believe,"* Ensign, May 2013, https://www.churchofjesuschrist.org/study/ensign/2013/05/sunday-afternoon-session/lord-i-believe?lang=eng

ACKNOWLEDGMENTS

Special thanks to my daughter, Emily, for her editing expertise. If there are faults in editing, they are mine because Emily helped so much when she could.

To those listed in Chapter 9, thank you for the hope you gave me during the difficulties of 2011. Support also looks like you!

I owe much gratitude to my memoir readers— Rick, Connie, Lil, Hunter, Sheri, Kim, Dana, Name Withheld 1 (who also contributed a story to chapter 10), and Name Withheld 2 (who also contributed a story to chapter 10).

Thanks to the others who contributed their personal stories in Chapter 10—Rick, Becky and Steve, Allen, Jared, Tom, Mae, and Mandy. Through your pain, we also saw your triumph!

Taryn, the Utah/Nevada Area Director of the American Foundation for Suicide Prevention, allowed my use of the Hope Squad hat in my picture and the AFSP materials for Chapter 11. Thank you so much!

So appreciative of my talented son Matt for the book cover design, his impressive picture of the Oregon coast, and the copy fitting.

I am eternally grateful to Heather Braley (LMFT), Debora Miller (LMFT), and Dr. Brian Goldman, MD—all gifted healers. Your guidance was invaluable. I owe you all so much!

ABOUT THE AUTHOR

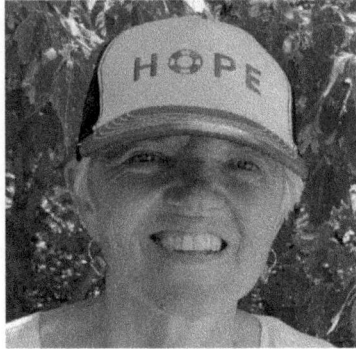

Jean Conley Stoddard is a Certified Mindfulness Meditation Instructor through the University of Holistic Theology—a fascinating distinction since, in 2011, she spent one month in three different mental hospitals diagnosed with clinical depression and anxiety. She recently became a Licensed Certified Substance Use Disorder Counselor.

Though it took many years, Jean did heal from her Category 5, Hurricane Katrina, storm-of-the-mind enabling her to share her fascinating story of what depression feels like from the inside out.

Jean indeed slogged through "the valley of the shadow of death" and came out the other side. Because she survived, she now shares that a depressed brain can heal and function even healthier than before. She emphatically declares, "There is hope!"

NOTE TAKING

www.ingramcontent.com/pod-product-compliance
Lightning Source LLC
Chambersburg PA
CBHW032133040426
42449CB00005B/219